Tittle

Nourishing Food Against Cancer

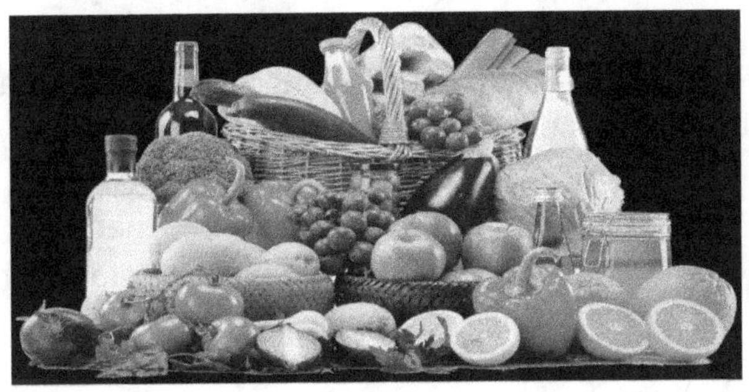

Subtitle

Cancer-Fighting Cuisine: Fuel for
Recovery

Webb Garza

Nourishing Food Against Cancer

Cancer-Fighting Cuisine: Fuel for Recovery

Introduction

Chapter 1

Understanding Cancer and Nutrition

(1.)Exploring the relationship between diet and cancer risk.

(2.)How certain foods and nutrients can contribute to prevention and healing.

(3.) The importance of balanced and wholesome eating patterns.

Chapter 2

Cellular Health Boost: The Synergistic Benefits of Vitamins, Minerals, Antioxidants, and Phytochemicals in Promoting Overall Well-being"

(1.)In-depth look at foods rich in vitamins A, C, E, selenium, and zinc with Examples.

(2.)The role of antioxidants in neutralizing harmful free radicals.

Chapter 3

Power of Plant-Based Foods

(1.)Advocating for a plant-centered diet and its benefits in cancer prevention.

(2.)Cancer-fighting compounds in vegetable

(3.)Recipes showcasing colorful, cancer-fighting meals.

Chapter 4

Healthy Fats for Protection

(1.)Exploring the role of omega-3 fatty acids and monounsaturated fats in reducing inflammation.

(2.) Discussing sources of healthy fats such as avocados, nuts, seeds, and fatty fish.

(3.) Tips for incorporating these fats into daily meals.

Chapter 5

Protein for Strength and Healing

(1.) Addressing the importance of lean protein sources in maintaining muscle mass during treatment.

(2.)Highlighting plant-based protein options and their benefits.

(3.)Sample meal plans that prioritize protein intake.

Chapter 6

Mindful Eating and Lifestyle

(1.)Discussing the impact of stress on cancer development and progression.

(2.)Exploring mindfulness techniques and stress-reducing practices.

(3.)Tips for cultivating a healthy relationship with food and promoting overall well-being.

Chapter 7

Use of Spices and Herbs in Food as Medicine

(1.)Showcasing the therapeutic properties of herbs and spices in cancer prevention.

(2.)examining the anti-inflammatory compounds in turmeric, ginger, garlic, and other herbs and spices provides insights into their potential health advantages. Let's delve into these ingredients and their impacts:

(3.) Creating dishes that incorporate these flavorful components.

Chapter 8

Staying Hydrated and Promoting Detoxification

(1.) Highlighting the significancep of maintaining cellular health through proper hydration.

(2.) Exploring the roles of water, herbal teas, and hydrating foods in maintaining hydration.

(3.) Dispelling misconceptions about extreme detox diets and advocating for balanced cleansing practices.

Chapter 9

Offering guidance on customizing your diet to your specific needs.

(1.) Providing guidance for individuals undergoing cancer treatment.

(2.).Addressing common dietary challenges during therapy.

(3.) Personalizing nutrition plans based on specific cancer types and stages.

Chapter 10

Building a Lifetime of Wellness

(1.) Approaches for Sustaining a Nourishing Diet Post-Treatment.

(2.) Encouraging Habits for Lifelong Well-Being and Vitality.

(3.)Sure, here are a couple of inspiring accounts of cancer survivors who reshaped their lives through changes in their eating habits:

Introduction

In a quiet town nestled between rolling hills, a story of resilience and hope unfolded. Emma, a spirited young woman, found herself facing the formidable adversary known as cancer. Fueled by her unwavering determination, Emma embarked on a journey to fight the disease with an unexpected ally – nourishing food.

Guided by her unyielding spirit, Emma delved into the world of nutrition and its potential to aid her battle. With the support of experts and her own research, she discovered the incredible power of certain foods to bolster her immune system and counteract the effects of treatment. Fruits bursting with antioxidants, vegetables teeming with vitamins, and whole grains brimming with vitality became her weapons.

As Emma's knowledge deepened, so did her connection with the community around her. Together, they planted gardens and shared recipes, cultivating a network of nourishment and camaraderie. The town's once-empty streets now echoed with the laughter of neighbors gathered around tables laden with vibrant, healthful dishes.

Emma's journey not only transformed her life but also ignited a spark of inspiration in others facing similar battles. Through her determination and the

magic of nourishing food, the town became a haven
of strength and resilience. Emma's story serves as
a testament to the profound impact that mindful
eating can have on the fight against cancer,
reminding us all that sometimes the simplest
ingredients yield the most extraordinary results.

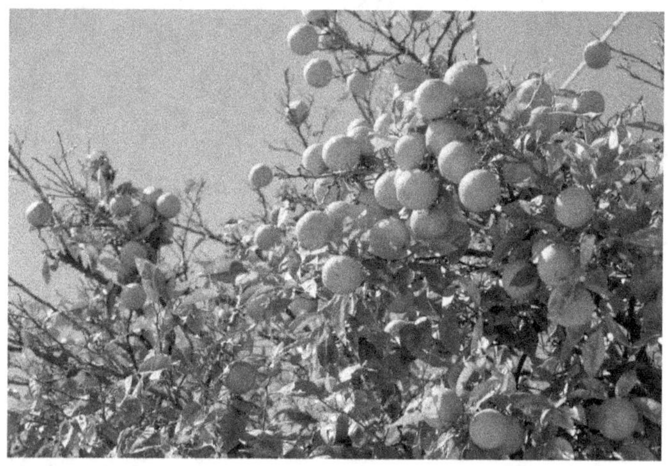

Chapter 1

Understanding Cancer and Nutrition

""Understanding the relationship between cancer and nutrition is crucial for overall health and well-being. While a healthy diet can't prevent cancer, it can play a significant role in reducing the risk and supporting treatment outcomes.

Certain dietary choices, such as consuming a variety of fruits, vegetables, whole grains, lean proteins, and healthy fats, can provide essential nutrients, antioxidants, and fiber that support the body's defense mechanisms against cancer. These nutrients help in reducing inflammation, supporting the immune system, and aiding in DNA repair.

On the other hand, a diet high in processed foods, sugary drinks, red and processed meats, and unhealthy fats may contribute to chronic inflammation and oxidative stress, increasing the risk of cancer development.

It's important to note that nutritional needs can vary depending on the type of cancer, stage of treatment, and individual health status. Cancer treatments like chemotherapy and radiation can have significant effects on appetite, taste perception, and nutrient absorption. Therefore, working with a registered dietitian who specializes in oncology can help develop personalized nutrition plans tailored to an individual's unique needs.

Maintaining a healthy weight is also crucial, as obesity is linked to a higher risk of certain types of cancer. Balancing calorie intake with physical activity is essential for weight management during and after cancer treatment.

In summary, a balanced and nutrient-rich diet can complement cancer treatment, enhance overall well-being, and potentially reduce the risk of cancer. Consulting with healthcare professionals can provide tailored guidance for maintaining proper nutrition throughout the cancer journey.

(1.)Exploring the relationship between diet and cancer risk.

**The intricate interplay between diet and cancer risk has garnered significant attention from researchers and health professionals alike. While genetics certainly play a role in cancer development, emerging evidence highlights the substantial influence that dietary choices exert on an individual's susceptibility to various types of cancer. This chapter delves into the multifaceted relationship between diet and cancer risk, shedding light on key mechanisms and factors that underscore this connection.

**1. **Understanding Carcinogenesis: At its core, cancer is characterized by the uncontrolled growth and spread of abnormal cells. Certain dietary patterns and specific nutrients can either promote or inhibit this process. The chapter will dissect how carcinogens and protective agents in foods can influence cellular mutations and DNA damage, contributing to the initiation and progression of cancer.

**2. **Inflammation and Immunity: Chronic inflammation has been recognized as a pivotal driver of cancer development. This section will delve into how certain dietary choices can trigger or alleviate inflammation, influencing the tumor microenvironment. Additionally, the impact of nutrition on the immune system's ability to detect and eliminate cancerous cells will be explored.

**3. **The Role of Oxidative Stress: The body's natural oxidation processes produce free radicals that can damage cellular structures and contribute to cancer risk. Antioxidants found in various foods serve as defense mechanisms against this oxidative stress. The chapter will discuss how a diet rich in antioxidants can help mitigate these damaging effects.

**4. **Hormones and Growth Factors: Hormones and growth factors play a pivotal role in cell growth and proliferation, and their disruption can contribute to cancer. Dietary choices can influence hormone levels and signaling pathways, potentially impacting cancer risk. This section will examine the connections between diet, hormones, and cancer development.

**5. **Weight Management and Obesity: Excess body weight is linked to an increased risk of several types of cancer. The chapter will explore how dietary habits contribute to weight gain and obesity, and how maintaining a healthy weight through balanced eating can lower the risk of cancer.

**6. **Specific Nutrients and Foods: Certain nutrients and bioactive compounds found in foods have been extensively studied for their potential in cancer prevention. This section will provide an overview of these substances, including vitamins, minerals, phytochemicals, and dietary fibers, and how they exert their protective effects.

**7. **Individualized Approaches: Recognizing that dietary needs and cancer risk factors vary from person to person, this chapter will emphasize the importance of personalized nutrition strategies. It will explore how factors like genetics, pre-existing health conditions, and lifestyle choices can influence an individual's response to different dietary interventions.

In deciphering the intricate connection between diet and cancer risk, individuals can make informed choices to reduce their susceptibility to this complex disease. Armed with a deeper understanding of the mechanisms at play, readers will be equipped to embark on a journey of healthier eating habits that have the potential to foster resilience and empower them in the fight against cancer.

(2.)How certain foods and nutrients can contribute to prevention and healing.

""Certain foods and nutrients play a significant role in both preventing and supporting the healing process of various health conditions, including cancer, cardiovascular diseases, diabetes, and more. Here are some examples:""

1. **Antioxidants**: Fruits and vegetables like berries, citrus fruits, leafy greens, and carrots are rich in antioxidants. These compounds help protect cells from damage caused by free radicals, potentially reducing the risk of chronic diseases and aiding in the healing process.

2. **Omega-3 Fatty Acids**: Found in fatty fish (salmon, mackerel, sardines), flaxseeds, and walnuts, omega-3 fatty acids have

anti-inflammatory properties that can aid in healing and reduce the risk of cardiovascular diseases.

3. **Fiber**: Foods like whole grains, legumes, fruits, and vegetables are high in dietary fiber. Adequate fiber intake supports digestive health, helps regulate blood sugar levels, and may lower the risk of certain cancers.

4. **Turmeric and Curcumin**: Turmeric contains curcumin, a compound known for its anti-inflammatory and antioxidant properties. It has been studied for its potential role in cancer prevention and as a complementary therapy in cancer treatment.

5. **Cruciferous Vegetables**: Broccoli, cauliflower, Brussels sprouts, and cabbage are rich in sulforaphane, a compound with potential anti-cancer properties. These vegetables may help in detoxification processes and support immune function.

6. **Vitamin D**: Sunlight exposure and certain foods (fatty fish, fortified dairy) provide vitamin D, which is essential for bone health and immune function. Some studies suggest it might play a role in reducing the risk of certain cancers.

7. **Green Tea**: Rich in catechins, green tea is believed to have antioxidant and anti-inflammatory

effects. Regular consumption has been associated with a reduced risk of certain types of cancer.

8. **Protein**: Lean protein sources like poultry, fish, beans, and lentils provide essential amino acids necessary for tissue repair and overall healing.

9. **Probiotics**: Yogurt, kefir, and fermented foods contain probiotics that support gut health and may aid in digestion, immune function, and even mental well-being.

10. **Zinc and Vitamin C**: These nutrients play a crucial role in wound healing, immune function, and collagen synthesis. Foods like citrus fruits, bell peppers, and nuts provide these nutrients.

Remember that a balanced diet with a variety of nutrient-rich foods is key. While certain foods and nutrients can contribute to prevention and healing, they should be part of an overall healthy lifestyle that includes regular physical activity, stress management, and avoiding overindulgence in processed foods, sweet snacks, and bad fats. It's always best to consult with healthcare professionals or registered dietitians for personalized guidance based on individual health needs and goals.

(3.) The importance of balanced and wholesome eating patterns.

Balanced and wholesome eating patterns are essential for maintaining optimal health, supporting physical well-being, and preventing various chronic diseases. Such eating patterns prioritize a variety of nutrient-rich foods in appropriate portions, offering a multitude of benefits:

1. **Nutrient Intake**: A balanced diet ensures that you receive a wide range of essential nutrients, vitamins, minerals, and antioxidants that your body needs for proper functioning, growth, and repair.

2. **Energy Levels**: Wholesome eating provides a steady supply of energy throughout the day. Balanced meals with carbohydrates, proteins, and healthy fats help stabilize blood sugar levels, preventing energy crashes and promoting sustained focus.

3. **Weight Management**: A balanced diet helps control calorie intake, which is crucial for weight management. It encourages consuming whole, unprocessed foods that are lower in empty calories and high in nutrients, making it easier to maintain a healthy weight.

4. **Digestive Health**: High-fiber foods such as whole grains, fruits, vegetables, and legumes

support digestion and prevent issues like constipation. A balanced diet also promotes a diverse gut microbiome, which is linked to better overall health.

5. **Heart Health**: A diet rich in fruits, vegetables, whole grains, lean proteins, and healthy fats (such as those from nuts, seeds, and fish) lowering blood pressure, inflammation, and cholesterol levels can help prevent heart disease.

6. **Bone Health**: Adequate calcium and vitamin D intake, which can be achieved through balanced eating, are crucial for maintaining strong bones and preventing osteoporosis.

7. **Cognitive Function**: Nutrient-rich foods, including those containing omega-3 fatty acids, antioxidants, and vitamins, are associated with better cognitive function and may help reduce the risk of cognitive decline as you age.

8. **Disease Prevention**: A balanced diet rich in fruits, vegetables, and whole grains is linked to a reduced risk of chronic diseases such as diabetes, certain cancers, and obesity.

9. **Mood and Mental Health**: Certain nutrients like B vitamins, magnesium, and omega-3 fatty acids are important for maintaining good mental health. A balanced diet can contribute to a positive

mood and may even help reduce the risk of
depression.

10. **Longevity**: Research suggests that adopting
a balanced and wholesome eating pattern can
contribute to a longer and healthier life.

Remember, balance is key. While it's important to
include a variety of nutrient-dense foods, it's also
okay to enjoy treats in moderation. Avoiding
extreme diets or severely restricting certain food
groups can help prevent nutrient deficiencies and
promote a sustainable approach to eating.

Ultimately, embracing a balanced and wholesome
eating pattern as part of an overall healthy lifestyle
is a powerful way to nourish your body, prevent
illness, and promote your well-being at every stage
of life.

Chapter 2

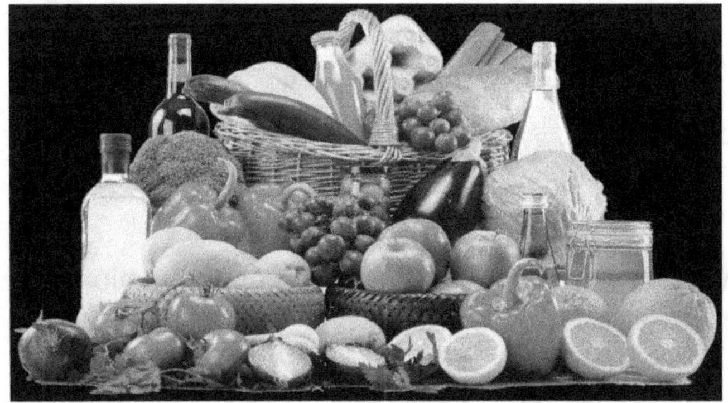

Cellular Health Boost: The Synergistic Benefits of Vitamins, Minerals, Antioxidants, and Phytochemicals in Promoting Overall Well-being"

These vitamins, minerals, antioxidants, and phytochemicals collectively contribute to cellular health by neutralizing harmful molecules, aiding in repair processes, and supporting various bodily functions. A balanced and diverse diet rich in these nutrients can go a long way in promoting the well-being of our cells and overall health.

(1.)In-depth look at foods rich in vitamins A, C, E, selenium, and zinc with Examples.

Vitamin A:
Vitamin A is crucial for vision, immune function, and skin health.
- **Sources:** Carrots, sweet potatoes, spinach, kale, butternut squash, apricots, and liver.

Vitamin C:
Vitamin C is a powerful antioxidant that supports the immune system, collagen production, and wound healing.
- **Sources:** Citrus fruits (oranges, grapefruits), strawberries, kiwi, bell peppers, broccoli, and Brussels sprouts.

Vitamin E:
Vitamin E is an antioxidant that protects cells from oxidative damage and supports skin health.
- **Sources:** Nuts (almonds, hazelnuts), seeds (sunflower seeds), spinach, broccoli, and vegetable oils (such as sunflower or olive oil).

Selenium:
Selenium is a mineral that supports antioxidant enzyme systems, thyroid function, and immune health.

- **Sources:** Brazil nuts (one of the richest sources), seafood (sardines, tuna), eggs, whole grains, and poultry.

Zinc:
Zinc is important for immune function, wound healing, and DNA synthesis.
- **Sources:** Oysters (highest zinc content), red meat, poultry, beans, nuts, and whole grains.

Incorporating these foods into your diet can help ensure you're getting an adequate intake of these essential nutrients. Remember, a diverse and balanced diet that includes a variety of fruits, vegetables, nuts, seeds, lean proteins, and whole grains will provide you with the vitamins, minerals, and antioxidants your body needs for optimal cellular health and overall well-being.

(2.)The role of antioxidants in neutralizing harmful free radicals.

Antioxidants play a crucial role in neutralizing harmful free radicals within the body, helping to maintain cellular health and prevent oxidative stress. Free radicals are unstable molecules with unpaired electrons that can damage cells, proteins, and DNA, potentially leading to various health issues and accelerating the aging process.

Antioxidants work by donating electrons to stabilize free radicals, thereby preventing them from causing further damage. Here are some examples of antioxidants and their role in neutralizing free radicals:

1. **Vitamin C (Ascorbic Acid):**
Vitamin C is a water-soluble antioxidant found in various fruits and vegetables. It helps protect cells and supports collagen production, immune function, and wound healing.

2. **Vitamin E (Tocopherols and Tocotrienols):**
Vitamin E is a fat-soluble antioxidant present in nuts, seeds, and vegetable oils. It helps protect cell membranes from oxidative damage and supports skin health.

3. **Beta-Carotene:**
Found in orange and yellow fruits and vegetables, as well as leafy greens, beta-carotene is converted into vitamin A in the body. It helps neutralize free radicals and supports vision and immune health.

4. **Selenium:**
Selenium is a mineral that serves as a component of antioxidant enzymes, such as glutathione peroxidase. It helps protect cells from oxidative stress and supports thyroid function.

5. **Flavonoids:**

Flavonoids are a group of phytochemicals found in colorful fruits, vegetables, tea, and cocoa. They have potent antioxidant and anti-inflammatory properties, contributing to overall cellular health.

6. **Lycopene:**
Lycopene is a red pigment found in tomatoes, watermelon, and other red and pink fruits. It's known for its antioxidant properties and potential role in reducing the risk of certain cancers.

7. **Quercetin:**
Present in apples, onions, and berries, quercetin is a flavonoid with antioxidant and anti-inflammatory effects, which may contribute to cardiovascular health.

By incorporating a variety of antioxidant-rich foods into your diet, you can help protect your cells from damage caused by free radicals. Remember that a balanced and diverse diet is essential for ensuring a sufficient intake of antioxidants and promoting overall health.

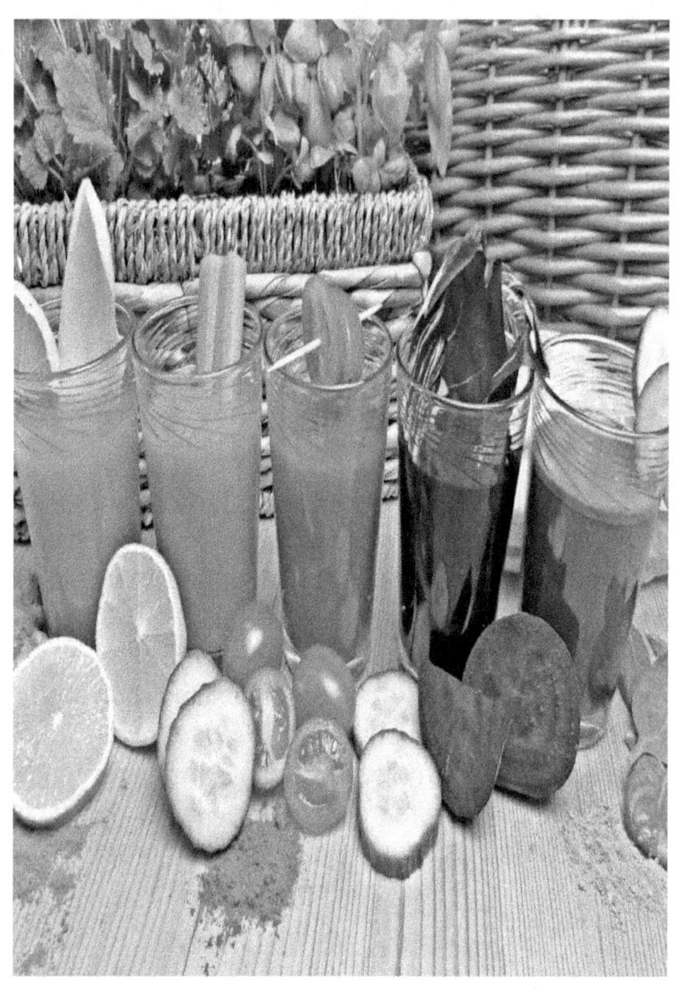

Chapter 3

Power of Plant-Based Foods

The power of plant-based foods lies in their ability to provide essential nutrients, promote health, and contribute to sustainability. Packed with vitamins, minerals, fiber, and phytochemicals, these foods support heart health, reduce the risk of chronic diseases, and offer diverse culinary options. Embracing plant-based choices can lead to improved well-being and a positive impact on the environment.

(1.)Advocating for a plant-centered diet and its benefits in cancer prevention.

Advocating for a plant-centered diet can significantly impact cancer prevention and overall well-being. Such a diet emphasizes the consumption of plant-based foods like fruits, vegetables, whole grains, legumes, nuts, and seeds, while minimizing the intake of animal products. The benefits of a plant-centered diet in cancer prevention are manifold:

1. **Antioxidant Richness:** Plant-based foods are naturally rich in antioxidants, which combat free radicals and reduce oxidative stress. This helps prevent DNA damage and reduces the risk of cancer development.

2. **Phytochemical Protection:** Plant foods contain phytochemicals like flavonoids, carotenoids, and glucosinolates, which possess anti-inflammatory and anticancer properties. They inhibit the growth of cancer cells and promote their destruction.

3. **Fiber Content:** A plant-centered diet is high in dietary fiber, which aids in digestion, maintains healthy gut bacteria, and regulates blood sugar levels. Fiber also helps prevent colorectal cancer by promoting regular bowel movements and removing toxins efficiently.

4. **Healthy Fats:** Nuts, seeds, and certain plant oils provide healthy fats that support cellular health and reduce inflammation. Omega-3 fatty acids found in flaxseeds and walnuts may also play a role in cancer prevention.

5. **Reduced Animal Products:** Limiting red and processed meats, often associated with an increased cancer risk, in favor of plant-based protein sources like beans, lentils, and tofu, can have a positive impact on cancer prevention.

6. **Weight Management:** A plant-centered diet tends to be lower in calories and saturated fats, which can contribute to maintaining a healthy weight. Excess body weight is a known risk factor for several types of cancer.

7. **Hormonal Balance:** Certain plant compounds, like phytoestrogens in soy products, can help regulate hormone levels. Balanced hormones are linked to a lower risk of hormone-related cancers such as breast and prostate cancer.

8. **Inflammation Reduction:** Chronic inflammation is associated with cancer development. Plant-based foods, rich in anti-inflammatory compounds, help reduce the body's inflammatory response.

9. **Gut Microbiome Health:** A diet rich in plant-based fiber supports a diverse and healthy gut microbiome, which plays a role in maintaining immune function and preventing inflammation-related cancers.

By adopting a plant-centered diet, individuals can empower themselves with a proactive approach to cancer prevention. However, it's essential to remember that a balanced and varied diet, along with a healthy lifestyle, contributes holistically to reducing cancer risk and supporting overall health.

(2.)Cancer-fighting compounds in vegetable

1.Certainly! One example of a cancer-fighting compound found in vegetables is sulforaphane. Sulforaphane is a natural compound that belongs to the family of isothiocyanates. It is particularly abundant in cruciferous vegetables such as broccoli, cauliflower, kale, and Brussels sprouts. Research suggests that sulforaphane may have anti-cancer properties due to its ability to support the body's detoxification processes, inhibit the growth of cancer cells, and reduce inflammation. Consuming these vegetables regularly may contribute to a lower risk of certain types of cancers.

2. **Vegetables:**
- **Glucosinolates (e.g., broccoli, cauliflower, cabbage):** These sulfur-containing compounds are found in cruciferous vegetables and are known for their potential anti-cancer properties, particularly in relation to digestive and hormone-related cancers.
- **Carotenoids (e.g., carrots, sweet potatoes, spinach):** Responsible for the orange, yellow, and green colors in vegetables, carotenoids like beta-carotene and lutein support eye health and may have antioxidant and immune-boosting effects.

3. **Legumes:**

- **Isoflavones (e.g., soybeans, lentils):** Found in soybeans and other legumes, isoflavones are known for their potential role in hormone regulation and reducing the risk of certain hormone-related cancers.
- **Phytic Acid (inhibitor of nutrient absorption):** While not necessarily a phytochemical with direct health benefits, phytic acid in legumes can bind to certain minerals and affect their absorption. Soaking, sprouting, or cooking legumes can help mitigate this.

4. **Whole Grains:**
- **Polyphenols (e.g., quinoa, oats, whole wheat):** Whole grains contain various polyphenols with antioxidant and anti-inflammatory properties that contribute to heart health and overall well-being.
- **Fiber (e.g., brown rice, whole wheat bread):** Although not a phytochemical, the fiber in whole grains supports digestive health, helps regulate blood sugar levels, and may contribute to a reduced risk of colorectal cancer.

Incorporating a colorful variety of these plant-based foods into your diet can provide a range of phytochemicals that work synergistically to promote health and potentially reduce the risk of chronic diseases, including certain types of cancer. Remember that a balanced diet rich in fruits, vegetables, legumes, and whole grains is essential for reaping the full benefits of these phytochemicals.

(3.)Recipes showcasing colorful, cancer-fighting meals.

Creating colorful, cancer-fighting meals can be both delicious and health-conscious. Incorporating a variety of fruits, vegetables, whole grains, and lean proteins can result in visually appealing dishes that are rich in phytochemicals and other nutrients. Here are a few recipe ideas:

1. **Rainbow Veggie Stir-Fry:**
A vibrant stir-fry that combines an array of colorful vegetables such as bell peppers (red, yellow, green), broccoli florets, carrots, and snap peas. Toss in lean protein like tofu or grilled chicken for a complete meal. The mix of colors indicates a range of phytochemicals, vitamins, and minerals that contribute to overall health.

2. **Mediterranean Quinoa Salad:**
Prepare a salad with cooked quinoa as the base. Add diced tomatoes (lycopene), cucumbers, red onions, bell peppers, and Kalamata olives. Feta cheese crumbles and olive oil are sprinkled on top. This salad showcases a blend of colors, providing antioxidants, fiber, and healthy fats.

3. **Berry Spinach Salad:**
Combine fresh baby spinach leaves with colorful berries like strawberries, blueberries, and raspberries (rich in anthocyanins). Add sliced almonds for crunch and grilled chicken or chickpeas for protein. Drizzle with a balsamic vinaigrette for a refreshing, cancer-fighting salad.

4. **Roasted Root Vegetables with Herbs:**
Roast a variety of root vegetables such as beets (betacyanins), sweet potatoes (beta-carotene), and rainbow carrots. Toss them with olive oil, fresh herbs like rosemary and thyme, and a sprinkle of sea salt. Roasting brings out the natural sweetness and enhances their cancer-fighting properties.

5. **Grilled Salmon with Mango Salsa:**
Grill a piece of wild-caught salmon and serve it with a vibrant mango salsa. Dice mangoes, red onions, bell peppers, and cilantro. Add a splash of lime juice and a touch of chili for flavor. The combination of omega-3 fatty acids in salmon and the antioxidants in mangoes creates a nutritious, flavorful dish.

6. **Tofu and Veggie Rainbow Wraps:**
Fill whole-grain wraps with grilled or sautéed tofu, a mix of colorful shredded veggies like red cabbage, carrots, and zucchini, and a drizzle of tahini or hummus. These wraps offer a variety of

textures and flavors along with cancer-fighting compounds.

Remember, the key is to incorporate a diverse range of colorful, whole foods into your meals. By doing so, you'll not only create visually appealing dishes but also provide your body with a spectrum of nutrients and antioxidants that can contribute to your overall health and potentially reduce the risk of cancer.

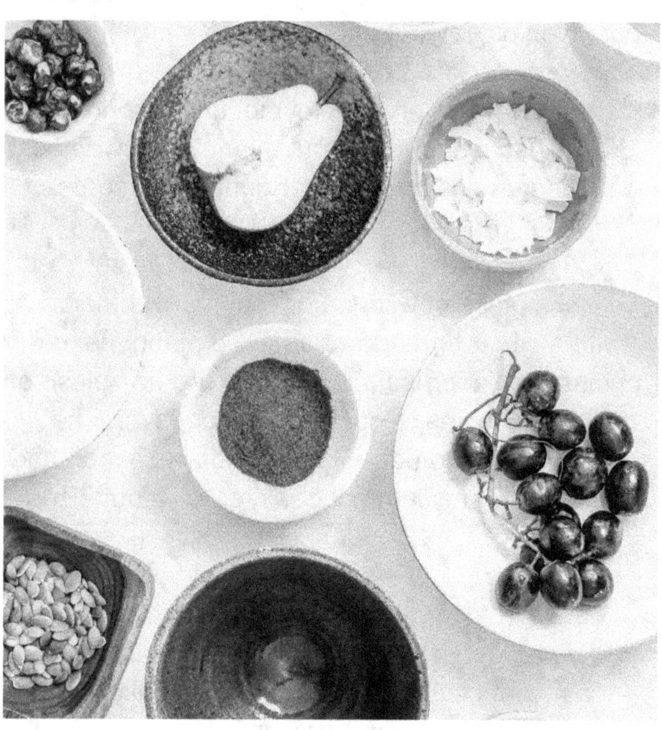

Chapter 4

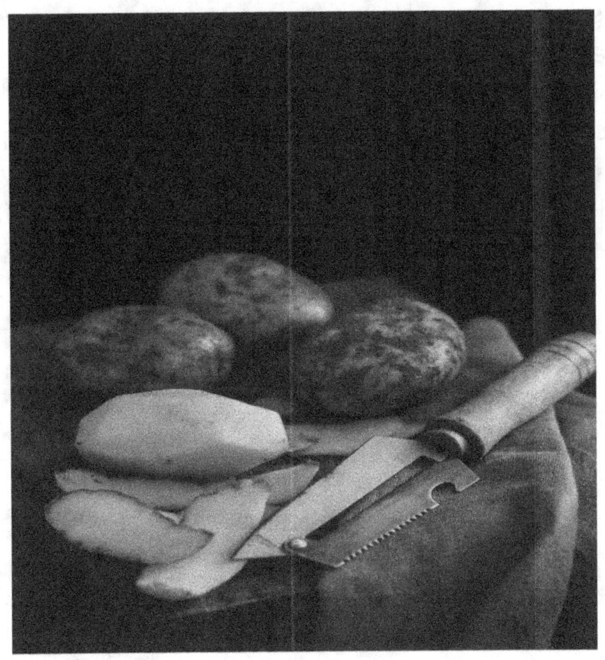

Healthy Fats for Protection

Healthy fats play a crucial role in protecting and supporting overall health. While it's important to limit saturated and trans fats, incorporating sources of healthy fats can provide a range of benefits for your body. Here are some examples of healthy fats and their protective properties:

1. **Monounsaturated Fats:**
Foods like avocados, olive oil, and nuts (almonds, pistachios) are rich in monounsaturated fats. These fats are known for their heart-protective effects by helping to lower bad cholesterol levels (LDL cholesterol) while maintaining or even increasing good cholesterol levels (HDL cholesterol). They also have anti-inflammatory properties, which can contribute to overall health.

2. **Polyunsaturated Fats:**
- **Omega-3 Fatty Acids:** Found in fatty fish (salmon, mackerel, sardines), flaxseeds, chia seeds, and walnuts, omega-3 fatty acids are essential for heart health. They have anti-inflammatory properties, support brain function, and may even help reduce the risk of chronic diseases like heart disease and certain types of cancer.
- **Omega-6 Fatty Acids:** These fats are present in sources like safflower, sunflower, and corn oils. While they are essential, the balance between omega-3 and omega-6 fatty acids is important. A diet high in omega-6 fatty acids and low in omega-3s can promote inflammation, so it's advisable to maintain a balanced intake.

3. **Coconut Oil:**
While it's debated among experts, coconut oil contains medium-chain triglycerides (MCTs) that are metabolized differently than other fats. Some

studies suggest that MCTs may have a neutral or even beneficial effect on heart health. However, due to its high saturated fat level, moderation is essential.

4. **Nuts and Seeds:**
Nuts and seeds like almonds, walnuts, chia seeds, and flaxseeds are packed with a combination of healthy fats, protein, fiber, and various vitamins and minerals. They provide sustained energy, support satiety, and offer protective effects for heart health.

5. **Avocado:**
Avocado is a nutrient-dense fruit that provides monounsaturated fats along with a host of vitamins, minerals, and fiber. Its fats contribute to better absorption of fat-soluble nutrients and may help reduce the risk of chronic diseases.

Incorporating these sources of healthy fats into your diet can help protect your body by promoting heart health, supporting brain function, and potentially reducing the risk of chronic diseases. Remember that moderation is key, as fats are calorie-dense, and a balanced diet that includes a variety of nutrients is essential for overall well-being.

(1.)Exploring the role of omega-3 fatty acids and monounsaturated fats in reducing inflammation.

Exploring the role of omega-3 fatty acids and monounsaturated fats in reducing inflammation reveals their significant impact on promoting overall health and well-being.

Omega-3 Fatty Acids:
Omega-3 fatty acids, found abundantly in fatty fish (such as salmon, mackerel, and sardines), flaxseeds, chia seeds, and walnuts, are renowned for their potent anti-inflammatory properties. These healthy fats are composed of two main types: eicosapentaenoic acid (EPA) and docosahexaenoic acid (DHA). They play a pivotal role in regulating the body's immune response and modulating inflammation.

Studies have shown that a diet rich in omega-3 fatty acids can help reduce the production of pro-inflammatory molecules, such as cytokines and prostaglandins. By doing so, omega-3s contribute to a decreased risk of chronic inflammatory conditions like cardiovascular disease, autoimmune disorders, and certain types of cancer. Additionally, these fats support brain health, helping to maintain cognitive function and potentially lowering the risk of neurodegenerative diseases.

Monounsaturated Fats:
Monounsaturated fats, present in foods like avocados, olive oil, and nuts, have been associated with a similar anti-inflammatory effect. They help balance the body's inflammatory responses by reducing the production of inflammatory markers.

Olive oil, in particular, contains a compound called oleocanthal, which has been likened to the anti-inflammatory effects of ibuprofen. This compound is believed to inhibit enzymes that trigger inflammation, making olive oil a valuable addition to an anti-inflammatory diet.

Incorporating omega-3 fatty acids and monounsaturated fats into your diet can lead to a healthier inflammatory balance in the body. By reducing chronic inflammation, you can help lower the risk of various chronic diseases and support your body's overall resilience. It's important to maintain a well-rounded diet that includes a variety of nutrient-rich foods to reap the full benefits of these healthy fats.

(2.) Discussing sources of healthy fats such as avocados, nuts, seeds, and fatty fish.

Sure, I'd be happy to discuss sources of healthy fats. Avocados, nuts, seeds, and fatty fish are all great examples. Monounsaturated fats, which are good for the heart, are abundant in avocados. which are heart-healthy fats. Nuts and seeds, like almonds, walnuts, chia seeds, and flaxseeds, provide a mix of healthy fats, fiber, and essential nutrients. Fatty fish such as salmon, mackerel, and sardines are high in omega-3 fatty acids, which are known for their anti-inflammatory properties and benefits for brain and heart health. Incorporating these foods into your diet can contribute to a balanced intake of healthy fats.

(3.) Tips for incorporating these fats into daily meals.

1. **Avocado Delights**:
- Spread mashed avocado on whole-grain toast and top it with a poached egg for a satisfying breakfast.
- Create a creamy avocado salad dressing by blending avocado, olive oil, lemon juice, and herbs.
- Add sliced avocado to your favorite wraps, sandwiches, or burgers for extra flavor and texture.

2. **Nutty and Seedy Goodness**:
- Mix a handful of almonds or walnuts into your morning yogurt or oatmeal.

- Sprinkle chia seeds or ground flaxseeds over smoothie bowls or cereal to boost omega-3 intake.
- Make your own trail mix with a variety of nuts, seeds, and a touch of dark chocolate for a healthy snack.

3. **Fish Feasts**:
- Grill or bake salmon fillets and serve them with a side of roasted vegetables for a balanced dinner.
- Create a colorful and nutritious salad by tossing together mixed greens, grilled mackerel, avocado slices, and a drizzle of olive oil.
- Enjoy canned sardines on whole-grain crackers as a quick and easy snack, or mix them into pasta dishes for added protein and flavor.

4. **Smart Cooking and Meal Prep**:
- Use olive oil or avocado oil for sautéing vegetables or as a base for marinades.
- Roast vegetables with a sprinkle of nuts or seeds to add crunch and healthy fats.
- Prepare a batch of homemade granola bars using nuts, seeds, and a bit of honey for a portable and nutritious snack.

5. **Balanced Combos**:
- Pair sliced avocado with grilled chicken in a wrap or sandwich for a satisfying lunch.
- Combine a handful of mixed nuts with fresh fruits for a balanced and energizing snack.
- Serve grilled fatty fish with a side of quinoa and steamed broccoli for a well-rounded dinner.

Remember, the key is to enjoy these healthy fats in moderation as part of a balanced diet. Mix and match these foods with a variety of other nutrient-rich ingredients to create meals that are both delicious and nourishing.

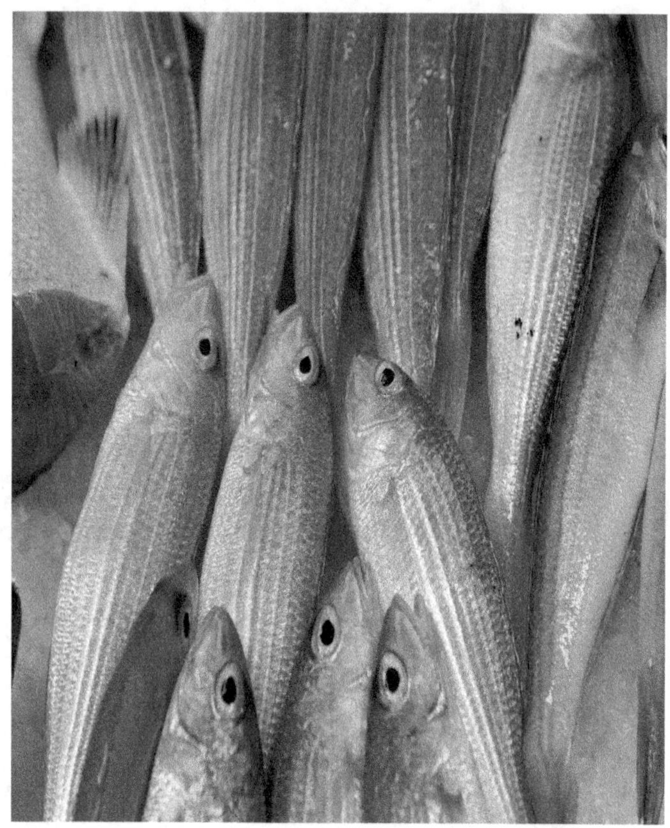

Chapter 5

Protein for Strength and Healing

Protein plays a crucial role in supporting both strength and healing within the body. Here's a breakdown of its importance in these areas:

1. Protein for Strength:
Protein is the building block of muscles. When you engage in physical activities such as strength training, your muscles experience microscopic damage. Protein helps repair and rebuild these muscle fibers, making them stronger and more resilient. Adequate protein intake is essential for individuals looking to increase muscle mass, improve athletic performance, or simply maintain their muscle health.

Examples of protein-rich foods for strength:
- Chicken, turkey, and lean beef cuts are examples of lean meats.
- Fish like cod, tuna, and salmon.
- Dairy items including low-fat milk, Greek yogurt, and cottage cheese.

- Plant-based options include quinoa, tofu, lentils, and beans.

2. Protein for Healing: Protein is also a critical component in the healing process. When the body undergoes injury or surgery, it requires additional protein to repair damaged tissues, support immune function, and promote wound healing. Protein contributes to the formation of collagen, a protein essential for repairing skin, tendons, ligaments, and other connective tissues.

Examples of protein-rich foods for healing:
- Eggs, which provide high-quality protein and essential amino acids.
- Nutrient-dense foods like nuts and seeds, which contain protein along with vitamins and minerals.
- Dairy or plant-based protein shakes can help meet increased protein needs during recovery periods.
- Lean meats and fish for a steady supply of amino acids that aid in tissue repair.

Remember, individual protein needs vary based on factors such as age, activity level, and health condition.Individualized advice can be obtained by contacting a licensed dietitian or healthcare provider. Incorporating a variety of protein sources into your diet ensures you receive a complete range of essential amino acids that contribute to both strength and healing.

(1.) Addressing the importance of lean protein sources in maintaining muscle mass during treatment.

Maintaining muscle mass during treatment is crucial for overall well-being and recovery. Lean protein sources play a significant role in this process due to their ability to provide essential nutrients and support muscle health. Here's why lean protein is essential and how it can help during treatment:

1. Preventing Muscle Loss:
Illness, medical treatments, and extended periods of inactivity can lead to muscle loss, known as muscle atrophy. Consuming adequate protein helps prevent this loss by providing the amino acids necessary for muscle maintenance and repair.

2. Supporting Recovery:
Medical treatments can put stress on the body, and recovery requires extra nutrients, including protein. Protein aids in wound healing, tissue repair, and immune system support, all of which are crucial during treatment.

3. Preserving Strength and Mobility:
Maintaining muscle mass contributes to better mobility, strength, and overall physical function.

This is especially important for patients who may experience weakness or fatigue due to treatment.

4. Optimizing Energy Levels:
Protein-rich foods provide a source of sustained energy. This is particularly valuable for patients who may be experiencing fatigue as a side effect of treatment.

5. Providing Essential Nutrients:
Lean protein sources, such as poultry, fish, legumes, and low-fat dairy, not only offer protein but also provide vitamins, minerals, and other nutrients that support overall health.

6. Meeting Nutritional Needs:
Treatment can sometimes affect appetite or taste preferences. Lean protein sources are often more palatable and easier to digest than fatty or heavy foods, making them a practical option to meet nutritional needs.

7. Personalized Nutrition:
Consulting a registered dietitian can help tailor protein intake to individual needs. They can provide recommendations based on treatment type, calorie needs, and dietary preferences.

Examples of lean protein sources:
- Skinless poultry (chicken, turkey)

- Fish (salmon, cod, tuna)
-Lean beef or pig chops that have been stripped of visible fat
- Low-fat dairy products (yogurt, milk)
- Legumes (beans, lentils)
- Tofu and tempeh
- Eggs and egg whites

Incorporating these lean protein sources into meals and snacks can help patients maintain muscle mass, support recovery, and improve overall well-being during treatment. It's important to work with healthcare professionals to develop a personalized nutrition plan that aligns with the specific treatment and health needs.

(2.)Highlighting plant-based protein options and their benefits.

Certainly, plant-based protein options offer a wealth of benefits for both your health and the environment. Here's a closer look at these options and their advantages:

1. Nutrient-Rich Choices:

Plant-based protein sources are often packed with vitamins, minerals, and dietary fiber. These nutrients contribute to overall health, digestion, and immune system function.

2. Heart Health:
Many plant-based proteins, such as beans, lentils, and nuts, are low in saturated fat and cholesterol. This makes them heart-healthy choices that can help lower the risk of cardiovascular diseases.

3. Weight Management:
Plant-based proteins are generally lower in calories and often high in fiber. This combination can help with weight management by promoting satiety and reducing overeating.

4. Reduced Environmental Impact:
Choosing plant-based proteins has a smaller environmental footprint compared to animal-based sources. Plant-based diets tend to require less land, water, and other resources, making them a more sustainable choice.

5. Lower Disease Risk:
A diet rich in plant-based proteins has been linked to a lower risk of chronic diseases such as type 2 diabetes, certain types of cancer, and hypertension.

6. Digestive Health:
Fiber is abundant in plant-based protein sources like legumes and whole grains. Fiber supports healthy digestion, aids in regular bowel movements, and may reduce the risk of digestive disorders.

7. Versatility:
Plant-based proteins can be incredibly versatile. You can use them in a wide variety of dishes, from salads and stir-fries to soups and stews.

8. Allergen-Friendly: For individuals with allergies or sensitivities to animal products, plant-based proteins offer an alternative that is free from common allergens like dairy and eggs.

Examples of plant-based protein sources and their benefits:

- **Legumes (Beans, Lentils, Chickpeas)**: Packed with protein, fiber, and various vitamins and minerals, legumes support digestion and contribute to steady energy levels.

- **Nuts and Seeds (Almonds, Chia Seeds, Sunflower Seeds)**: Rich in healthy fats, protein, and essential nutrients, nuts and seeds are excellent for heart health and brain function.

- **Tofu and Tempeh**: Soy-based products that provide complete protein and can be used in a variety of dishes. They are also sources of calcium and iron.

- **Quinoa**: A complete protein source containing all nine essential amino acids, quinoa is also gluten-free and high in fiber.

- **Seitan**: A protein-rich wheat gluten product often used as a meat substitute in vegetarian and vegan diets.

- **Plant-Based Dairy Alternatives (Soy Milk, Almond Milk)**: Fortified plant-based milks protein and are suitable alternatives for those who are lactose intolerant or choose to avoid dairy.

Incorporating these plant-based protein sources into your diet can bring about positive health benefits while contributing to a more sustainable and environmentally-friendly way of eating. Remember to create balanced meals that include a variety of protein sources to ensure you're getting all the essential amino acids your body needs.

(3.)Sample meal plans that prioritize protein intake.

Of course, here are a few sample meal plans that prioritize protein intake while incorporating a variety of foods for balanced nutrition:

Sample Meal Plan 1: Balanced Breakfast, Lunch, and Dinner

Breakfast:
- Scrambled tofu with sautéed vegetables (bell peppers, spinach, onions, tomatoes).
- Whole-grain toast.
- A small serving of mixed berries.

Lunch:
- Chickpea salad with mixed greens, cherry tomatoes, cucumbers, and red onions.
- Quinoa (cooked) as a base.
- Drizzle of olive oil and lemon juice for dressing.

Dinner:
- Baked salmon fillet seasoned with herbs and lemon.
- Steamed broccoli and roasted sweet potatoes.

- Mixed beans (black beans, kidney beans) sautéed with garlic and a touch of olive oil.

Snacks:
- Greek yogurt with a sprinkle of almonds and chia seeds.
- Carrot and celery sticks with hummus.

Sample Meal Plan 2: Plant-Based Protein Focus

Breakfast:
- Overnight oats made with rolled oats, almond milk, chia seeds, and a scoop of plant-based protein powder.

- Sliced banana and a drizzle of almond butter on top.

Lunch:
- Lentil soup with plenty of vegetables (carrots, celery, spinach).
- A side of quinoa or whole-grain bread.

Dinner:- Grilled tofu skewers marinated in a teriyaki sauce. - Stir-fried mixed vegetables (broccoli, bell peppers, snap peas) with garlic and ginger.

- Brown rice as a base.

Snacks:
- Handful of mixed nuts (almonds, walnuts) and dried apricots.
- Apple slices with peanut butter.

Sample Meal Plan 3: High-Protein Options

Breakfast:
- Scrambled eggs with diced bell peppers, onions, and spinach.
- Whole-grain English muffin.

Lunch:
- Grilled chicken breast slices over a bed of mixed greens.
- Quinoa salad with chopped cucumbers, tomatoes, and a light vinaigrette dressing.

Dinner:
- Lean beef stir-fry with broccoli, snow peas, and carrots in a soy-ginger sauce.
- Cauliflower rice.

Snacks:
- Cottage cheese with sliced strawberries.

- Rice cakes topped with hummus and sliced turkey.

Remember, these meal plans are just examples and can be adjusted based on your individual dietary preferences, calorie needs, and any specific nutritional goals you have. To ensure you're meeting your protein intake needs, consider consulting a registered dietitian or nutritionist who can provide personalized guidance tailored to your requirements.

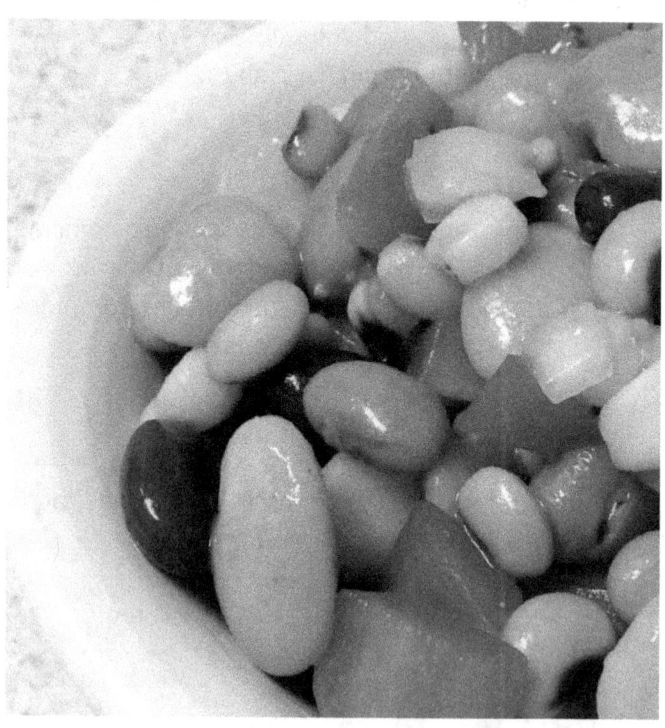

Chapter 6

Mindful Eating and Lifestyle

Mindful eating is a practice that involves paying full attention to the experience of eating and drinking, both in terms of the food itself and the sensations that arise during the process. It encourages being present in the moment, engaging all the senses, and fostering a deeper connection with the act of nourishing oneself.

Incorporating mindful eating into your lifestyle can have several benefits. It helps prevent overeating by promoting awareness of hunger and fullness cues, which can support weight management. By savoring each bite, you might find a greater appreciation for the flavors and textures of your food. This approach can lead to a more positive relationship with eating and reduce the tendency to use food as a way to cope with emotions.

To practice mindful eating, start by sitting down at a table without distractions like phones or TVs. Take a few deep breaths to center yourself before beginning to eat. As you eat, focus on the taste, smell, and texture of the food. Chew slowly and pay attention to the sensations in your body as you swallow. Notice any thoughts or judgments that arise about the food, and let them go without attaching to them.

Incorporating mindfulness into other aspects of your lifestyle, such as daily activities and interactions, can also lead to a more balanced and fulfilling life. Mindfulness practices like meditation and yoga can complement mindful eating, fostering an overall sense of well-being. Remember, the goal isn't perfection but rather an increased awareness of your choices and actions.

Overall, adopting a mindful approach to both eating and lifestyle can help you cultivate a greater sense of awareness, gratitude, and harmony in your daily life.

(1.)Discussing the impact of stress on cancer development and progression.

Certainly. Stress is a complex physiological and psychological response that can have a significant impact on various aspects of our health, including cancer development and progression. While the exact mechanisms are not fully understood, research suggests that chronic stress may play a role in influencing cancer in several ways.

1. **Immune Suppression:** Prolonged stress can lead to a suppressed immune system, impairing the body's ability to detect and control the growth of cancer cells. This weakened immune response might make it easier for cancer cells to evade the body's defense mechanisms.

2. **Inflammation:** Chronic stress triggers inflammation in the body, which is believed to be a contributing factor in cancer development and progression. Inflammatory processes can create an environment that supports tumor growth and spread.

3. **Hormonal Changes:** Stress activates the release of stress hormones like cortisol and adrenaline. These hormones can affect various cellular processes and disrupt the body's hormonal balance. High levels of stress hormones over time might create conditions that favor cancer growth.

4. **Angiogenesis:** Stress might promote the growth of new blood vessels (angiogenesis), which is essential for tumors to grow beyond a certain size. Angiogenesis supplies tumors with nutrients and oxygen, facilitating their expansion.

5. **DNA Damage:** Stress-induced oxidative stress can lead to DNA damage, potentially increasing the likelihood of mutations that contribute to cancer development. Unrepaired DNA

damage can result in the formation of cancerous cells.

6. **Behavioral Factors:** Chronic stress can lead to unhealthy coping behaviors like smoking, excessive alcohol consumption, poor diet, and lack of physical activity. These behaviors are known to be risk factors for cancer.

7. **Treatment Response:** Stress may also affect how a person responds to cancer treatments. High stress levels can impact a patient's ability to tolerate treatment side effects and may influence treatment outcomes.

It's important to note that while stress can potentially influence cancer, it is just one of many factors. Genetic predisposition, environmental exposures, lifestyle choices, and overall health also play crucial roles in cancer development and progression.

Managing stress through strategies like mindfulness, meditation, regular exercise, and seeking support from friends, family, or professionals can be beneficial not only for general well-being but also potentially for reducing the impact of stress on cancer-related processes. However, stress reduction should be considered as a complementary approach to cancer management, in addition to medical treatments prescribed by healthcare professionals.

(2.)Exploring mindfulness techniques
and stress-reducing practices.

Certainly, exploring mindfulness techniques and stress-reducing practices can greatly contribute to overall well-being and help manage the challenges of modern life. Here are some practical methods to take into account:

1. **Mindful Breathing:** One of the simplest and most powerful mindfulness practices is focusing on your breath. Take a few minutes to sit quietly, close your eyes, and bring your attention to your breath. Feel the sensation of each inhale and exhale, letting go of any distractions.

2. **Body Scan Meditation:** In this practice, you systematically bring your awareness to different parts of your body, noticing any sensations without judgment. This can help you become more attuned to bodily sensations and release tension.

3. **Meditation:** Engage in regular meditation sessions to cultivate mindfulness. You can begin with a small amount of time each day and progressively increase the amount of time. There are various types of meditation, including focused

attention, loving-kindness, and body-centered practices.

4. **Yoga:** Yoga combines physical postures with breath awareness, promoting relaxation and flexibility. It can help release physical tension and create a sense of calm.

5. **Mindful Eating:** As discussed earlier, mindful eating involves savoring each bite, paying attention to the flavors, textures, and sensations of eating.This may result in better eating patterns and a happier relationship with food.

6. **Nature Walks:** Spending time in nature and observing your surroundings mindfully can be incredibly soothing. Pay attention to the colors, sounds, and textures around you as you take a leisurely walk.

7. **Progressive Muscle Relaxation:** This technique involves tensing and then releasing different muscle groups in your body. It helps you become aware of muscle tension and learn how to relax it.

8. **Journaling:** Writing down your thoughts and feelings can provide an outlet for stress and help you gain insights into your emotions. You can also jot down things you're grateful for each day.

9. **Deep Breathing Exercises:** Practice deep, slow breathing to activate the body's relaxation response. Breathe in deeply through your nose, pause for a moment, and then slowly let out through your mouth.

10. **Guided Imagery:** Close your eyes and imagine a peaceful and calming scene, engaging your senses to create a vivid mental image. This can transport you to a serene mental space.

11. **Mindful Technology Use:** Be conscious of how you use technology. Take breaks from screens, and consider using mindfulness apps or features that remind you to pause and breathe.

12. **Setting Boundaries:** Learn to say no when you're feeling overwhelmed. Establishing boundaries in your personal and professional life can help manage stress.

Remember that practicing mindfulness and stress reduction is a journey, and what works best for one person may not work the same way for another. It's important to find techniques that resonate with you and integrate them into your daily routine. Consistency is key, and over time, these practices can lead to a greater sense of calm, focus, and resilience in the face of stress.

(3.)Tips for cultivating a healthy relationship with food and promoting overall well-being.

Cultivating a healthy relationship with food is essential for promoting overall well-being. Here are some tips to help you establish a positive and balanced approach to eating:

1. **Practice Mindful Eating:** Eat with awareness and pay attention to your hunger and fullness cues. Engage all your senses in the experience of eating to truly savor and appreciate your meals.

2. **Avoid Restrictive Diets:** Instead of following strict diets, focus on incorporating a variety of whole, nutrient-dense foods into your diet. Balance is key.

3. **Listen to Your Body:** Learn to recognize your body's signals for hunger and satiety. Eat when you're hungry and stop when you're comfortably full.

4. **Eat Intuitively:** Trust your body to guide your food choices. Honor your cravings and preferences without guilt.

5. **Practice Moderation:** Allow yourself to enjoy your favorite treats in moderation. This can help prevent feelings of deprivation and binge eating.

6. **Meal Planning:** Plan balanced meals and snacks ahead of time to avoid making impulsive and unhealthy choices when hungry.

7. **Stay Hydrated:** Drink enough water throughout the day to support your body's functions and maintain energy levels.

8. **Include Fiber:** Incorporate fiber-rich foods like whole grains, fruits, vegetables, and legumes to support digestion and keep you feeling satisfied.

9. **Mindful Portioning:** Be mindful of portion sizes to prevent overeating. You can use visual cues like your hand or smaller plates to help with portion control.

10. **Cook at Home:** Preparing meals at home gives you more control over ingredients and allows you to enjoy cooking as a creative and mindful activity.

11. **Avoid Emotional Eating:** Find alternative ways to cope with emotions, such as going for a walk, practicing deep breathing, or journaling.

12. **Practice Self-Compassion:** Be kind to yourself and avoid negative self-talk. Remember that one indulgence won't derail your overall health journey.

13. **Regular Physical Activity:** Engage in regular exercise that you enjoy. Physical activity contributes to overall well-being and can help you feel more in tune with your body.

14. **Seek Professional Help:** If you're struggling with disordered eating patterns or a negative relationship with food, consider seeking support from a registered dietitian or mental health professional.

15. **Celebrate Non-Food Achievements:** Recognize that your worth and accomplishments extend beyond food choices. Celebrate your achievements and qualities that have nothing to do with your appearance or what you eat.

16. **Educate Yourself:** Learn about the nutritional value of different foods and how they contribute to your well-being. Knowledge can empower you to make informed choices.

Remember that cultivating a healthy relationship with food takes time and patience. It's a journey of self-discovery, self-care, and self-compassion. By adopting these tips and approaching food with a positive mindset, you can nourish your body, mind, and soul for a happier and healthier life.

Chapter 7

Use of Spices and Herbs in Food as Medicine

Since ancient times, culinary herbs and spices have been used to enhance the flavor of food as well as for possible therapeutic purposes. These organic ingredients are full of a variety of bioactive substances that have positive health effects. Here are some typical culinary spices and herbs along with some potential medical applications:

1.**turmeric**Turmeric has anti-inflammatory and antioxidant properties and is best known for its active ingredient, curcumin. It's often used to support joint health, reduce inflammation, and aid digestion.

2.Ginger:** Ginger contains gingerol, which has anti-inflammatory, antioxidant, and nausea-reducing properties. It helps to support the immune system, ease muscle pain, and treat digestive problems.

3. **Gladiator:** Allicin, a substance in garlic with antimicrobial and immune-stimulating properties.It's believed to support heart health by reducing cholesterol levels and blood pressure.

4. **Cinnamon:** Cinnamon has anti-inflammatory properties and is high in antioxidants. It might enhance insulin sensitivity, control blood sugar levels, and promote brain health.

5. **Oregano:** Oregano contains compounds like carvacrol with antimicrobial properties. It's used to boost the immune system and support respiratory health.

6. **Rosemary:** Rosemary contains rosmarinic acid and antioxidants. It's believed to enhance cognitive function, support digestion, and have anti-inflammatory effects.

7. **Basil:** Basil contains essential oils like eugenol with antimicrobial properties. It is used as a digestive aid and may have anti-inflammatory properties.

8. **Thyme:** Thymol, an ingredient in thyme, has antioxidant and antimicrobial properties. It's used to support respiratory health and boost the immune system.

9. **Peppermint:** Peppermint contains menthol, known for its soothing effects on digestion. It's used to alleviate gastrointestinal discomfort and support respiratory health.

10. **Cayenne Pepper:** Cayenne contains capsaicin, which has pain-relieving and

metabolism-boosting properties. It may support weight management and help alleviate pain.

11. **Coriander:** Coriander contains antioxidants and may have antimicrobial properties. It's used to support digestion and may help manage blood sugar levels.

12. **Sage:** Sage contains compounds like rosmarinic acid with antioxidant and anti-inflammatory effects. It's believed to support cognitive health and soothe sore throats.

It's important to understand that while culinary herbs and spices may have health benefits, they shouldn't be used in place of medical care. Including a variety of herbs and spices in your diet can improve your overall health, but it's best to speak with a doctor before using any of them as remedies, especially if you have underlying medical issues or are taking prescription drugs.

Cooking with these savory and aromatic ingredients can not only make your meals more exciting but also possibly improve your health in a number of ways.

(1.)Showcasing the therapeutic properties of herbs and spices in cancer prevention.
Although culinary herbs and spices cannot replace medical treatments, recent research indicates that some of the compounds present in these natural

ingredients may have potential advantages in cancer support and prevention. Here are some herbs and spices that have demonstrated positive therapeutic effects in this situation:

1.**turmeric** The active ingredient in turmeric, curcumin, has received extensive research regarding its ability to reduce inflammation and to act as an antioxidant. It might aid in promoting apoptosis (cell death) and reducing the growth of cancer cells. According to research, curcumin may be able to stop or slow the growth of a number of cancer types.

2.** garlic** Organosulfur compounds found in garlic have been linked to anti-cancer properties. These substances could facilitate the activation of enzymes that detoxify carcinogens and inhibit the development oftumor cells. Consuming garlic has been associated with a lower risk of developing some cancers, including colorectal and stomach cancer.

3. **Ginger:** Gingerol, found in ginger, has demonstrated anti-inflammatory and antioxidant effects. According to some research, ginger extract may slow the growth of cancer cells and reduce nausea and vomiting brought on by chemotherapy.

4.** Cruciferous vegetables (brussels sprouts, cauliflower, and broccoli)**: These vegetables contain sulforaphane and indole-3-carbinol, substances that may have cancer-preventing qualities but are neither spices or herbs. They might aid in detoxifying and stop the spread of cancerous cells.

5.** Rosemary** Both the rosmarinic acid and the carnosic acid found in rosemary have anti-inflammatory and antioxidant effects. These substances may aid in preventing DNA damage and limiting the development of some cancer cells, according to some study.

6.**Cinnamon** The main ingredient in cinnamon, cinnamonaldehyde, has demonstrated anti-inflammatory and antioxidant properties. There has to be more research, however some studies indicate that cinnamon may help stop the spread of cancer cells.

7. **Thyme:** Thymol and carvacrol found in thyme have demonstrated antioxidant and antimicrobial properties. These compounds might contribute to thyme's potential cancer-preventive effects.

It's worth mentioning that although these herbs and spices have displayed promising outcomes in lab and animal research, more extensive investigation is required to fully grasp their potential in preventing and treating cancer. Furthermore, their effects can differ based on factors like dosage, personal health conditions, and interactions with other drugs.

If you're considering adding these herbs and spices to your diet for possible cancer prevention, it's advisable to do so as part of a well-rounded eating plan. Always consult a healthcare expert before making significant dietary adjustments or using herbs and spices as a form of therapy, especially if you have a cancer history or other medical issues.

(2.)examining the anti-inflammatory compounds in turmeric, ginger, garlic, and other herbs and spices provides insights into their potential health advantages. Let's delve into these ingredients and their impacts:

1. **Turmeric (Curcumin):** Curcumin, the primary bioactive component in turmeric, possesses strong anti-inflammatory properties. It suppresses molecules involved in inflammation, potentially reducing chronic inflammation tied to various health conditions. Additionally, it aids in generating antioxidants, which can further counter inflammation.

2. **Ginger (Gingerol):** Gingerol, the main bioactive compound in ginger, has potent anti-inflammatory effects by inhibiting the production of inflammatory molecules. It might also decrease oxidative stress and regulate immune responses, contributing to its anti-inflammatory attributes.

3. **Garlic (Organosulfur Compounds):** Garlic contains organosulfur compounds such as allicin, which hold anti-inflammatory properties. These compounds can regulate the immune system and diminish inflammation, particularly beneficial for cardiovascular health.

4. **Cinnamon (Cinnamaldehyde):** Cinnamaldehyde, responsible for cinnamon's unique flavor, displays anti-inflammatory effects by inhibiting the release of pro-inflammatory molecules. Additionally, its antioxidant properties contribute to its potential to combat inflammation.

5. **Rosemary (Rosmarinic Acid and Carnosic Acid):** Rosemary features rosmarinic acid and carnosic acid, both with anti-inflammatory properties. These compounds might suppress the activation of inflammatory enzymes and lower oxidative stress, leading to overall anti-inflammatory effects.

6. **Thyme (Thymol and Carvacrol):** Thymol and carvacrol are key active compounds in thyme. Their antioxidant and anti-inflammatory properties are well-studied, inhibiting inflammatory molecule production and safeguarding against oxidative damage.

7. **Oregano (Carvacrol):** Carvacrol, a primary oregano compound, demonstrates anti-inflammatory effects. It can influence

inflammatory pathways and potentially alleviate inflammation-related symptoms.

8. **Basil (Eugenol):** Eugenol, found in basil, exhibits anti-inflammatory properties by reducing the production of inflammatory molecules and supporting immune function.

9. **Peppermint (Menthol):** Menthol in peppermint exhibits anti-inflammatory effects by curbing the production of inflammatory cytokines. It offers relief from various inflammatory conditions, especially those affecting digestion.

These anti-inflammatory compounds target different pathways in the inflammatory response. Chronic inflammation is linked to health issues like heart disease, diabetes, and certain cancers. Integrating these herbs and spices into your diet could contribute to an anti-inflammatory eating plan, potentially lowering the risk of chronic diseases and promoting overall well-being.

Remember, while these compounds show anti-inflammatory effects in studies, they are just one part of a holistic health approach. Prior to making significant dietary changes or using herbs and spices for therapeutic reasons, especially if you have existing health conditions or take medications, consult a healthcare professional.

(3.) Creating dishes that incorporate these flavorful components.

Absolutely! Here are some culinary ideas that infuse the vibrant and anti-inflammatory herbs and spices we've discussed:

1. **Radiant Turmeric Smoothie:**
- Ingredients: 1 cup almond milk, 1 frozen banana, 1 tsp turmeric powder, ½ tsp ginger powder, ¼ tsp cinnamon, 1 tbsp chia seeds.
- Instructions: Blend all ingredients until velvety. Adjust the spice levels to your liking. The turmeric and ginger lend an anti-inflammatory warmth to this luscious smoothie.

2. **Roasted Vegetables with Garlic and Herbs:**
- Ingredients: Assorted vegetables (e.g., carrots, bell peppers, zucchini, broccoli), minced garlic, fresh rosemary and thyme, olive oil, salt, pepper.
- Instructions: Toss veggies with olive oil, minced garlic, and fresh herbs. Roast until tender. The garlic and herbs infuse flavor and anti-inflammatory goodness.

3. **Ginger-Garlic Sautéed Delight:**
- Ingredients: Lean protein (chicken, tofu, shrimp), mixed veggies (bell peppers, broccoli, snap peas), minced ginger and garlic, low-sodium soy sauce.
- Instructions: Sauté protein and veggies with minced ginger and garlic. Add a splash of soy sauce for flavor. The ginger and garlic inject an

anti-inflammatory twist into this swift and delectable
stir-fry.

4. **Cinnamon-Spiced Morning Bliss:**
- Ingredients: Rolled oats, almond milk, sliced
bananas, ground cinnamon, chopped nuts, honey
or maple syrup.
- Instructions: Cook oats in almond milk and top
with sliced bananas, a sprinkle of ground
cinnamon, chopped nuts, and a drizzle of honey or
maple syrup. The cinnamon not only imparts
warmth but also anti-inflammatory benefits.

5. **Rosemary and Thyme Grilled Chicken:**
- Ingredients: Chicken breasts, fresh rosemary
and thyme, olive oil, lemon juice, salt, pepper.
- Instructions: Marinate chicken with olive oil,
lemon juice, chopped rosemary, thyme, salt, and
pepper. Grill to perfection. The rosemary and thyme
infuse aromatic flavors and potential
anti-inflammatory effects.

6. **Basil and Tomato Delight:**
- Ingredients: Fresh tomatoes, fresh basil leaves,
extra-virgin olive oil, balsamic vinegar, salt, pepper,
mozzarella (optional).
- Instructions: Layer tomatoes with fresh basil
leaves. Drizzle with olive oil and balsamic vinegar,
and season with salt and pepper. Add mozzarella if
desired. Basil's sweet aroma adds a burst of
freshness and potential anti-inflammatory
advantages.

Remember, adapt these recipes to suit your tastes and dietary requirements. Introducing these herbs and spices into your meals can elevate not just the taste but also the potential health gains. Always seek guidance from a healthcare professional for any specific health concerns or dietary constraints before making significant dietary changes.

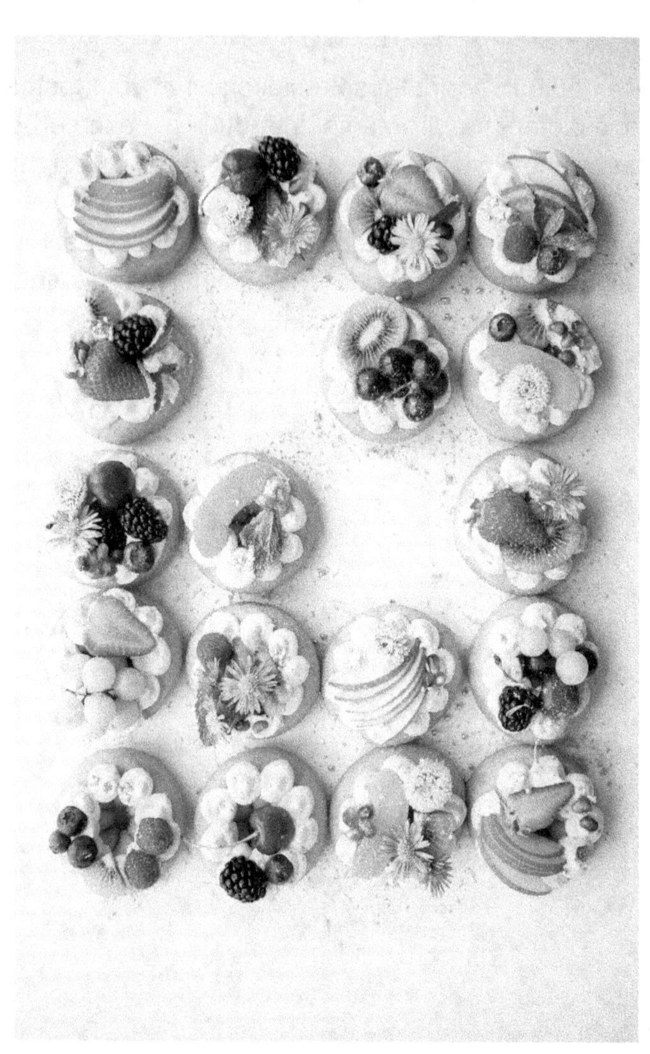

Chapter 8

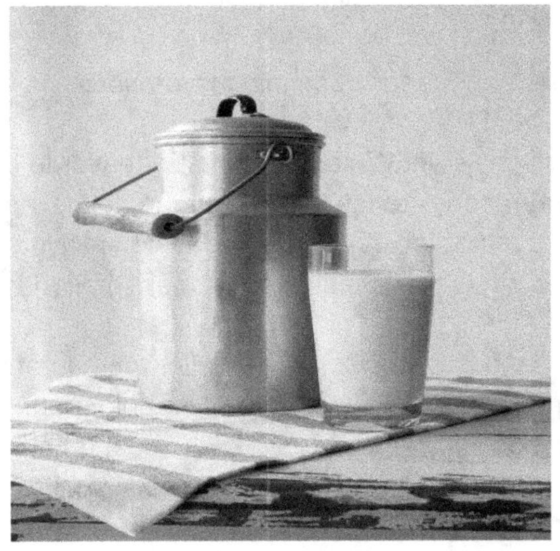

Staying Hydrated and Promoting Detoxification

Maintaining hydration and promoting detoxification are pivotal for upholding a robust body and fostering overall well-being. Let's explore these aspects more comprehensively:

Staying Hydrated:
Hydration pertains to providing your body with ample fluids to sustain its regular functions. Water is essential for diverse bodily processes, encompassing digestion, circulation, temperature control, and waste elimination. Optimal hydration supports ideal bodily operations and bolsters overall health.

Tips for Sustaining Hydration:

1. **Consistent Water Intake:** Endeavor to drink water consistently throughout the day, even if you're not feeling thirsty. Delaying until you're thirsty might indicate mild dehydration.

2. **Assess Urine Color:** Monitor the hue of your urine. A pale yellow or light straw color generally signifies sufficient hydration, while darker shades may indicate the need for more fluids.

3. **Include Hydrating Foods:** Incorporate foods with high water content, such as fruits (watermelon, oranges, cucumbers) and vegetables (lettuce, celery, bell peppers).

4. **Restrict Dehydrating Drinks:** Limit consumption of beverages that could lead to dehydration, like sugary drinks and excessive caffeine.

5. **Factor in Electrolytes:** If you engage in vigorous physical activity or experience significant sweating, contemplate consuming beverages with added electrolytes to replenish lost minerals.

Detoxification:
Detoxification refers to the body's process of eliminating or neutralizing toxins and waste products. Natural detoxification systems, including the liver, kidneys, and digestive system, function to expel harmful substances. While certain advocates propose specific detox diets or products, the body's inherent detox mechanisms are typically proficient on their own.

Tips for supporting natural detoxification:

1. **Healthy Diet:** Consume a diet rich in fruits, vegetables, whole grains, lean proteins, and healthy fats. These provide essential nutrients that support the body's detoxification processes.

2. **Stay Hydrated:** Drinking enough water helps flush toxins out of the body through urine and sweat.

3. **Physical Activity:** Regular exercise supports circulation and helps the body eliminate waste products.

4. **Adequate Fiber Intake:** Fiber aids digestion and helps eliminate waste from the intestines.

Whole grains, fruits, and vegetables are excellent sources of fiber.

5. **Limit Processed Foods:** Minimize the consumption of processed foods high in added sugars, unhealthy fats, and additives that might burden the body's detoxification systems.

6. **Mindful Eating:** Pay attention to portion sizes and eat mindfully to avoid overeating, which can strain digestion and metabolism.

7. **Adequate Sleep:** Quality sleep allows the body to repair and regenerate, supporting its natural detoxification processes.

It's important to approach detoxification in a balanced and evidence-based manner. Extreme detox diets or cleanses that involve severe caloric restriction or extreme fasting can have negative consequences for overall health. Always consult with a healthcare professional before making significant changes to your diet or engaging in detoxification programs, especially if you have underlying health conditions.

(1.) Highlighting the significancep of maintaining cellular health through proper hydration.

Proper hydration is crucial for supporting cellular health and overall well-being. Every cell in your body requires water to function effectively, and maintaining adequate hydration ensures that essential cellular processes occur seamlessly. Here's why underscoring the importance of hydration is key for cellular health:

1. Nutrient Transportation:
Water serves as a medium for delivering nutrients to cells. It conveys vital vitamins, minerals, and electrolytes to cells, facilitating their growth, repair, and overall function. Inadequate hydration can compromise nutrient supply to cells, impacting their vitality.

2. Elimination of Waste:
Cells produce waste products as part of various metabolic activities. Water plays a critical role in flushing out these waste materials from cells and the body. Proper hydration ensures efficient waste removal, preventing the accumulation of toxins that can hinder cellular function.

3. Cellular Communication:
Cells communicate through chemical signals that rely on water. Sufficient hydration supports the

transmission of these signals, facilitating proper coordination and functioning of different types of cells.

4. Enzymatic Reactions:
Enzymes, which drive biochemical reactions, require a water-rich environment to function optimally. Enzymes play a pivotal role in cellular metabolism, energy production, and other essential processes. Inadequate hydration can impede enzymatic reactions, leading to cellular dysfunction.

5. Temperature Regulation:
Water helps regulate body and cellular temperatures. Cells perform best within a narrow temperature range. Maintaining proper hydration assists in preserving this balance, preventing cells from becoming too hot or cold.

6. Cellular Structure and Form:
Water provides structural support to cells, maintaining their shape and integrity. Cells deprived of adequate water can become shrunken and less effective in performing their functions.

7. Electrolyte Equilibrium:
Electrolytes like sodium, potassium, and chloride are vital for maintaining cellular balance and electrical potential. Adequate hydration helps regulate these electrolytes, ensuring that cells retain their electrical properties for optimal function.

8. DNA Replication and Protein Synthesis:
Water is essential for DNA replication and protein synthesis, fundamental processes driving cell division and growth. Hydration creates the necessary environment for these complex biochemical reactions.

9. Oxygen Transport:
Water is a critical component of blood, which transports oxygen from the lungs to cells throughout the body. Well-hydrated cells receive an ample supply of oxygen, promoting efficient cellular respiration and energy production.

10. Overall Cellular Well-being:
Hydrated cells are more resilient and better equipped to handle stress. Proper hydration supports the body's ability to repair damaged cells, promoting the overall health and longevity of cells.

Incorporating healthy hydration habits into your daily routine is crucial to ensure that your cells operate optimally. Keep in mind that individual hydration requirements can vary based on factors like age, activity level, and climate. Paying attention to your body's thirst signals and consistently drinking water is a simple yet powerful way to prioritize cellular health and support the countless processes within your body's cells.

(2.) Exploring the roles of water, herbal teas, and hydrating foods in maintaining hydration.

Certainly! Water, herbal teas, and hydrating foods all play vital roles in maintaining hydration and supporting overall well-being. Let's delve into their importance:

Water:
Water serves as the foundation of hydration and is essential for various bodily functions. Here's why water is crucial:

1. **Cellular Function:** Water facilitates the transport of nutrients to cells and the removal of waste products from cells. It supports cellular communication, enzymatic reactions, and overall cellular health.

2. **Temperature Regulation:** Water helps regulate body temperature, preventing overheating during physical activity or in hot conditions.

3. **Digestion and Absorption:** Water aids in digesting and absorbing nutrients. It supports the function of digestive enzymes and the movement of food through the digestive tract.

4. **Joint Lubrication:** Adequate hydration helps lubricate joints, promoting smooth movement and reducing discomfort.

5. **Skin Health:** Proper hydration maintains skin elasticity, preventing dryness and promoting a healthy complexion.

Herbal Teas:
Herbal teas offer flavorful and hydrating alternatives to plain water. Many herbal teas also provide additional health benefits:

1. **Hydration:** Herbal teas are primarily composed of water, making them an effective way to increase fluid intake.

2. **Antioxidants:** Some herbal teas, such as green tea and hibiscus tea, are rich in antioxidants that combat oxidative stress and contribute to overall health.

3. **Digestive Support:** Herbal teas like peppermint and ginger tea can aid digestion, alleviate discomfort, and reduce bloating.

4. **Relaxation and Stress Relief:** Chamomile and lavender teas possess calming properties that help reduce stress and promote relaxation.

5. **Anti-Inflammatory Effects:** Turmeric and ginger teas contain anti-inflammatory compounds that may support overall well-being.

Hydrating Foods:
Certain foods with high water content contribute to hydration:

1. **Fruits:** Water-rich fruits like watermelon, cucumber, oranges, and berries provide hydration and essential vitamins.

2. **Vegetables:** Vegetables like lettuce, celery, and zucchini are primarily composed of water and offer additional nutrients.

3. **Soups and Broths:** Soups and broths made with water-based ingredients provide both hydration and nourishment.

4. **Smoothies:** Blending hydrating fruits and vegetables into smoothies is an excellent way to increase fluid intake while enjoying a nutrient-rich beverage.
5. **Yogurt and Cottage Cheese:** These dairy products contain water and provide protein and calcium.

Incorporating a mix of water, herbal teas, and hydrating foods into your daily routine is a comprehensive approach to maintaining hydration. Remember that individual hydration needs vary based on factors like age, activity level, and climate. Listening to your body's cues of thirst and consuming a variety of hydrating options will help ensure that you maintain optimal hydration levels for overall health and well-being.

(3.) Dispelling misconceptions about extreme detox diets and advocating for balanced cleansing practices.

Certainly, extreme detox diets often promise quick and dramatic results but can be misleading and potentially harmful. Let's debunk common myths about extreme detox diets and emphasize the importance of balanced cleansing practices:

Myth 1: Extreme Detox Diets Provide Quick Solutions:
Fact: Extreme detox diets promising rapid weight loss or complete body "cleansing" tend to be unsustainable and may result in short-term outcomes followed by weight regain.

Myth 2: Detox Diets Completely Eliminate Toxins:
Fact: The body has natural detoxification mechanisms, primarily managed by the liver, kidneys, skin, and lungs. Detox diets cannot entirely remove toxins, and extreme approaches

may even disrupt the body's natural detox processes.

Myth 3: Severe Calorie Restriction is Beneficial:
Fact: Drastically cutting calories through extreme detox diets can deprive the body of essential nutrients, leading to nutrient deficiencies, muscle loss, and a slowed metabolism.

Myth 4: Weight Loss Equals Detoxification:
Fact: Weight loss does not directly indicate detoxification. Many extreme detox diets lead to water and muscle loss rather than toxin elimination.

Myth 5: Herbal Supplements Ensure Safe Detox:
Fact: Some detox diets include herbal supplements claiming to aid detoxification. However, the safety and effectiveness of such supplements are often not well-reg

Chapter 9

Offering guidance on customizing your diet to your specific needs.

Customizing your diet according to your individual requirements is a crucial step in optimizing your health and well-being. The nutritional needs of each person are distinct and influenced by factors like age, gender, activity level, health status, and personal preferences. Here's how you can personalize your diet to best suit your needs:

1. Define Your Goals:
Clearly identify your health objectives. Are you aiming for weight management, enhanced energy levels, better digestion, muscle gain, or something else? Having clear goals will guide your dietary choices.

2. Consider Your Lifestyle:
Factor in your daily routine, work schedule, physical activity level, and eating habits. This information will help shape a diet that is both practical and sustainable for you.

3. Acknowledge Dietary Restrictions:

If you have dietary restrictions or allergies, ensure these are central to your considerations. Focus on obtaining all essential nutrients while avoiding foods that trigger adverse reactions.

4. Understand Nutrient Requirements:
Different life stages necessitate varying nutrients. For instance, growing children, pregnant or breastfeeding individuals, and seniors have unique nutritional needs. Research the vital nutrients for your age and life stage.

5. Opt for Whole Foods:
Prioritize whole, minimally processed foods. These foods deliver essential nutrients in their natural forms, contributing to overall well-being.

6. Balance Macronutrients:
Determine the ideal balance of carbohydrates, proteins, and fats based on your goals. Athletes or those engaging in intense training might require more carbohydrates, while those aiming for weight loss could benefit from increased protein intake.

7. Prioritize Micronutrients:
Vitamins and minerals are essential for various bodily functions. Create meals that incorporate a variety of colorful fruits and vegetables to ensure a diverse range of micronutrients.

8. Adjust Caloric Intake:

Your calorie needs depend on factors like age, gender, activity level, and objectives. Calculate your daily caloric requirements and adapt your intake accordingly.

9. Listen to Your Body:
Pay attention to signals of hunger and fullness. Eat when hungry and stop when satisfied. This mindful approach can prevent overeating and support digestion.

10. Experiment and Adapt:
Individual responses to foods vary. Experiment with different foods and meal timings to determine what works best for your body. Be open to making adjustments as needed.

11. Stay Hydrated:
Monitor your fluid intake and adjust it based on activity levels and climate. Hydration is essential for overall health.

12. Seek Expert Advice:
If you're uncertain about how to tailor your diet effectively, consider consulting a registered dietitian or nutritionist. They can offer personalized recommendations based on your needs and goals.

Remember, there's no universal diet that suits everyone. Customizing your diet involves finding a balance that aligns with your objectives and promotes your overall well-being. It's an ongoing process that requires self-awareness, flexibility, and a commitment to prioritizing your health.

(1.) Providing guidance for individuals undergoing cancer treatment.

Certainly, individuals undergoing cancer treatment require specialized care and attention to support their health and well-being. While the specifics of guidance can vary based on the type of cancer and treatment plan, here are some general suggestions to consider:

1. Communication with Healthcare Team:
Maintain open and regular communication with your oncologist and healthcare team. They can provide personalized advice, monitor your progress, and address any concerns or side effects.

2. Balanced Nutrition:
Eating a well-balanced diet is crucial. Focus on whole foods, lean proteins, whole grains, fruits, vegetables, and healthy fats. Proper nutrition can support your immune system, energy levels, and overall healing process.

3. Hydration:
Stay hydrated by drinking enough water throughout the day. Proper hydration can help manage side effects and support bodily functions.

4. Manage Side Effects:
Cancer treatments often come with side effects like nausea, fatigue, and changes in appetite. Work with your healthcare team to manage these symptoms through medications, dietary adjustments, and other supportive strategies.

5. Protein Intake:
Adequate protein intake is important for tissue repair and immune function. Include sources like lean meats, poultry, fish, eggs, dairy products, legumes, and nuts.

6. Nutrient-Dense Foods:
Choose nutrient-dense foods to provide your body with essential vitamins and minerals. Incorporate a variety of colorful fruits and vegetables for antioxidants and other beneficial compounds.

7. Small, Frequent Meals:
If you're experiencing appetite changes, consider eating smaller, more frequent meals throughout the day to help maintain your energy levels.

8. Avoid Excessive Sugar and Processed Foods:
Limit sugary foods and beverages, as well as highly processed items. These choices can negatively impact energy levels and overall health.

9. Be Cautious with Supplements:

Consult your healthcare team before taking any supplements, as some might interfere with your treatment or have unintended side effects.

10. Listen to Your Body:
Pay attention to how your body responds to different foods and adjust your diet accordingly. If certain foods are causing discomfort or worsened side effects, consider avoiding them temporarily.

11. Physical Activity:
Engage in gentle physical activities that are appropriate for your energy levels and treatment plan. Consult your healthcare team before starting any exercise regimen.

12. Emotional Support:
Seek emotional support through counseling, support groups, or spending time with loved ones. Emotional well-being is an integral part of your overall health.

13. Rest and Sleep:
Prioritize rest and quality sleep. Adequate sleep supports the body's healing processes and helps manage fatigue.

14. Maintain Social Connections:
Stay connected with friends and family. Social support can have positive effects on your mental and emotional well-being.

15. Mindfulness and Stress Reduction:
Practice relaxation techniques, mindfulness, and stress reduction strategies. These practices can help manage anxiety and promote a sense of calm.

Remember that every individual's journey with cancer is unique. What works for one person might not work for another. Work closely with your healthcare team to create a personalized plan that addresses your specific needs, treatment plan, and goals. Their expertise and guidance will play a crucial role in helping you navigate through this challenging time.

(2.).Addressing common dietary challenges during therapy.

While undergoing cancer therapy, individuals frequently encounter various dietary obstacles due to treatment side effects and shifts in appetite. Overcoming these obstacles is pivotal to ensuring that patients receive sufficient nourishment to bolster their overall well-being and recovery. Here are typical dietary challenges and strategies for managing them:

1. Nausea and Vomiting:

Challenge: Chemotherapy and radiation often lead to nausea and vomiting, which can impede eating.

Strategies:

- Opt for mild, bland foods that are less likely to trigger nausea.
- Consume smaller, frequent meals throughout the day.
- If hot foods trigger discomfort, choose cold or room temperature options.
- Stay hydrated by sipping clear fluids between meals.

2. Changes in Taste and Smell:

Challenge: Cancer treatment can distort taste and smell, causing appetite loss or aversion to certain foods.

Strategies:

- Experiment with diverse flavors and textures to identify what's more appealing.
- Enhance taste with seasonings like herbs, spices, and lemon.
- If meat is unpalatable, try alternative protein sources like eggs, tofu, beans, and lentils.

3. Mouth Sores and Swallowing Difficulty:

Challenge: Mouth sores and swallowing troubles can make eating painful.

Strategies:

- Opt for soft, easily swallowable foods such as yogurt, pureed soups, mashed potatoes, and smoothies.

- Avoid spicy, crunchy, or acidic foods that may
exacerbate mouth discomfort.
- Use a recommended salt and baking soda
solution to rinse your mouth.

4. Fatigue:
Challenge: Cancer therapy fatigue can diminish
energy for meal preparation and consumption.
Strategies:
- Opt for simple, quick-to-make meals and snacks.
- Cook and store meals ahead of time during
periods of higher energy.
- Seek assistance from family, friends, or caregivers
in meal preparation.

5. Diarrhea or Constipation:
Challenge: Some cancer treatments can lead to
diarrhea or constipation, affecting digestion.
Strategies:
- Gradually increase fiber intake to promote
balanced bowel movements.
- Stay hydrated to counter dehydration due to
diarrhea.
- For constipation, consume fiber-rich foods and
ample water.

6. Loss of Appetite:
Challenge: Reduced appetite is frequent during
cancer treatment, leading to diminished food intake.
Strategies:
- Consume small, nutrient-dense meals and snacks
across the day.

- Prioritize calorie-rich foods like nuts, seeds, avocados, and nut butters.
- Experiment with food and meal timings to determine effective approaches.

7. Weight Changes:
Challenge: Cancer treatment can result in weight loss or gain, impacting overall health.
Strategies:
- Collaborate with a registered dietitian to create a balanced meal plan supporting energy needs and health goals.
- Emphasize nutrient-rich foods for essential vitamins and minerals.

8. Dehydration:
Challenge: Certain therapies, such as chemotherapy, can cause dehydration.
Strategies:
- Regularly consume water, herbal teas, and clear broths.
- Opt for hydrating foods like watermelon, oranges, and cucumbers.

9. Food Safety:
Challenge: Weakened immunity during treatment increases susceptibility to foodborne infections.
Strategies:
- Avoid raw or undercooked foods, unpasteurized dairy, and deli meats.

- Thoroughly wash fruits and vegetables, and adhere to proper food handling and hygiene.

Effective communication with your healthcare team and a registered dietitian is crucial to addressing specific dietary challenges faced during cancer treatment. They offer personalized counsel and tailored recommendations, ensuring adequate nutrition to support healing and overall well-being.

(3.) Personalizing nutrition plans based on specific cancer types and stages.

Customizing nutrition plans to align with distinct cancer types and stages is pivotal in optimizing treatment outcomes, managing side effects, and bolstering overall health. Varied cancers and stages elicit differing nutritional needs and considerations. Here's how nutrition plans can be uniquely tailored to specific cancer types and stages:

Breast Cancer:

Early Stage:
- Emphasize a balanced diet rich in whole grains, lean proteins, healthy fats, fruits, and vegetables.
- Maintain a healthy weight to mitigate recurrence risks.
- Monitor bone health through calcium and vitamin D sources.

- Limit processed foods and alcohol in favor of whole alternatives.

Advanced Stage:
- Adequate protein intake supports muscle retention.
- Consider calcium and vitamin D for sustained bone health.
- Address weight fluctuations for optimal well-being.

Colorectal Cancer:

Pre-Surgery (Neoadjuvant):
- Prioritize high-fiber foods for digestive health and regular bowel movements.
- Stay hydrated to combat constipation.
- Focus on protein to preserve muscle strength prior to surgery.

Post-Surgery (Adjuvant):
- Gradually reintroduce fiber after surgery to alleviate discomfort.
- Protein and nutrient intake are critical for post-surgery wound healing.
- Address hydration and side effects such as diarrhea or constipation.

Lung Cancer:

Early and Advanced Stages:
- Prioritize balanced nutrition for overall health and immune support.

- Adequate protein supports healing and muscle preservation.
- Monitor weight fluctuations for enhanced treatment outcomes.

Prostate Cancer:

Early and Advanced Stages:
- Opt for a diet abundant in fruits, vegetables, whole grains, and healthy fats.
- Include foods beneficial for prostate health, such as tomatoes (high in lycopene), omega-3 fatty acids, and cruciferous vegetables.
- Manage weight, aiming for optimal body composition.

Gastric (Stomach) Cancer:

Pre-Surgery (Neoadjuvant):
- Focus on balanced nutrition for overall strength prior to surgery.
- Address weight changes for sustained nourishment.

Post-Surgery (Adjuvant):
- Opt for smaller, more frequent meals to manage potential appetite shifts.
- Prioritize easily digestible nutrient-rich foods.
- Hydration contributes to digestion and overall health.

Remember, these are general guidelines. Tailored recommendations from a registered dietitian or healthcare professional consider factors like medical history, treatment plan, allergies, side effects, and personal preferences. Cancer treatment nutrition aims to cater to unique needs, fostering health and quality of life. Prior to substantial dietary changes or new food or supplement additions, always consult your healthcare team.

Chapter 10

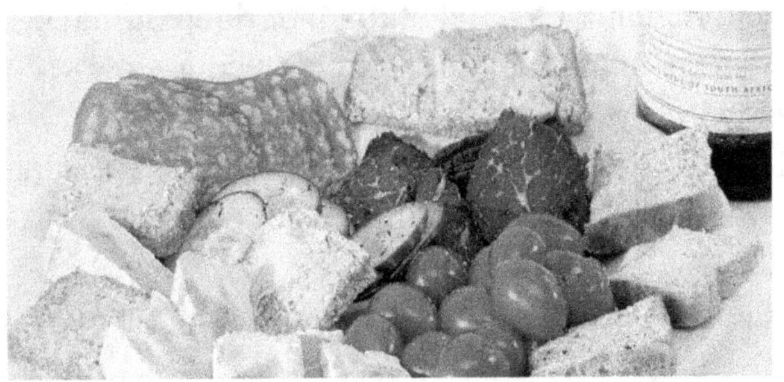

Building a Lifetime of Wellness

Creating a lifelong journey of wellness involves consistently making positive choices that bolster your physical, mental, and emotional well-being. It's about adopting healthy habits and practices that enrich your quality of life and empower you to flourish. Here's how you can construct a lifetime of wellness:

1. Prioritize Physical Well-Being:
- Regularly engage in physical activities you enjoy, such as walking, dancing, swimming, or yoga.
- Embrace a balanced diet abundant in whole foods, lean proteins, fruits, vegetables, and whole grains.
- Ensure adequate sleep to facilitate your body's repair and renewal processes.

2. Cultivate Mental and Emotional Wellness:
- Utilize mindfulness, meditation, or deep breathing techniques to manage stress and encourage relaxation.
- Give prominence to self-care endeavors that bring joy, whether it's reading, hobbies, or spending time outdoors.
- Foster a positive outlook and practice gratitude.

3. Nourish Strong Relationships:
- Establish and sustain healthy relationships with friends, family, and your community.
- Communicate openly and attentively to nurture meaningful connections.

4. Lifelong Learning:
- Participate in continual learning to keep your mind engaged and inquisitive.
- Embark on new hobbies, pick up a musical instrument, learn a language, or enroll in educational classes.

5. Stay Socially Engaged:
- Partake in social activities and gatherings to remain linked with others and counteract feelings of isolation.

6. Regular Health Assessments:
- Arrange routine health checkups and screenings to detect potential health concerns early.

7. Embrace Gratitude:
- Foster an attitude of gratitude by focusing on the positive facets of your life.

8. Develop Resilience:
- Foster resilience to navigate obstacles and setbacks with a constructive mindset.

9. Set Practical Goals:
- Establish attainable goals that contribute to your general well-being and celebrate your accomplishments.

10. Connect with Nature:
- Dedicate time outdoors to recharge and establish a connection with the natural world.

11. Limit Screen Exposure:
- Set boundaries on screen time to prevent excessive digital consumption and promote face-to-face interactions.

12. Volunteer and Contribute:
- Engage in volunteer activities that serve your community and provide a sense of purpose.

13. Manage Stress:
- Cultivate healthy coping mechanisms, such as exercise, hobbies, or relaxation techniques, to handle stress.

14. Cultivate Positivity:

- Foster a positive perspective on life by concentrating on solutions instead of problems.

15. Enjoy Laughter and Fun:
- Infuse laughter and enjoyment into your daily routine to elevate mood and alleviate stress.

Keep in mind that building a lifelong journey of wellness is an individualized process. What suits one person may not work for another, making it crucial to heed your body's signals and prioritize practices that make you feel your best. Implement gradual shifts and commemorate achievements along the way. Ultimately, the aim is to create a comprehensive approach to wellness that bolsters your physical, mental, and emotional health throughout the years.

(1.) Approaches for Sustaining a Nourishing Diet Post-Treatment.

Maintaining a nourishing diet following cancer treatment is pivotal for aiding recovery, managing potential side effects, and sustaining overall well-being. Here are strategies to consider as you transition to a healthy and balanced diet post-treatment:

1. Gradual Transition:

Ease into dietary changes step by step. Begin by reintroducing foods that were restricted during treatment, while being attuned to your body's response. Pay heed to your body's cues and adjust as necessary.

2. Prioritize Whole Foods:
Concentrate on nutrient-rich whole foods that supply vital vitamins, minerals, and antioxidants. Opt for an assortment of fruits, vegetables, lean proteins, whole grains, and healthy fats.

3. Hydration:
Continue to stay hydrated by consuming ample water throughout the day. Adequate hydration supports digestion, energy levels, and overall bodily functions.

4. Balanced Meals:
Opt for balanced meals that incorporate a mix of protein, healthy fats, and complex carbohydrates. This equilibrium aids in stabilizing blood sugar levels and furnishing sustained energy.

5. Emphasis on Fiber:
Integrate fiber-rich foods like whole grains, legumes, fruits, and vegetables. Fiber promotes digestive health, assists in maintaining a healthy weight, and offers a sensation of fullness.

6. Portion Management:

Be attentive to portion sizes to avoid overindulgence. Utilizing smaller plates and bowls can facilitate portion regulation.

7. Minimize Processed Foods:
Limit intake of highly processed foods high in added sugars, unhealthy fats, and sodium. Choose fresh, minimally processed alternatives whenever feasible.

8. Address Digestive Changes:
In the presence of digestive issues, consider consuming smaller, more frequent meals to prevent discomfort. Integrate foods that are gentle on digestion, such as cooked vegetables and lean proteins.

9. Manage Weight Changes:
If your weight altered during treatment, collaborate with a registered dietitian to devise a healthful eating strategy aligned with your current goals and supportive of weight management.

10. Incorporate Antioxidants:
Include foods teeming with antioxidants, like berries, leafy greens, nuts, and seeds. Antioxidants shield cells from damage and boost overall well-being.

11. Tackle Taste Changes:
If taste alterations persist, experiment with diverse flavors and textures to discover what is appealing.

Augment the taste of your meals with herbs, spices, and citrus.

12. Maintain Physical Activity:
Participate in regular physical activities you enjoy. Exercise bolsters overall health, elevates energy levels, and enhances mental well-being.

13. Regular Health Checkups:
Persist in scheduling regular health checkups and screenings to monitor progress and address any concerns.

14. Seek Guidance from a Dietitian:
Engaging with a registered dietitian specializing in oncology can yield tailored counsel attuned to your distinct needs and inclinations.

15. Embrace Mindful Eating:
Consume mindfully, savoring each bite and paying heed to hunger and satiety cues. Mindful eating promotes sound digestion and a favorable relationship with food.

Remember that post-treatment nutrition is an expedition demanding patience and self-care. Your body has undergone significant changes, necessitating nourishment with compassion and understanding. By implementing these strategies, you can buttress recovery and embrace a nourishing diet conducive to overall well-being.

(2.) Encouraging Habits for Lifelong Well-Being and Vitality.

Urging habits that champion lifelong well-being and vitality is an impactful means of investing in your health and savoring an enriched quality of life. These habits empower you to feel invigorated, resilient, and equipped to confront life's trials. Here are pivotal habits to adopt for enduring health and vitality:

1. Elevate Balanced Nutrition:
Consume a medley of nutrient-packed foods, encompassing fruits, vegetables, lean proteins, whole grains, and healthy fats. Strive for a well-rounded diet that furnishes essential vitamins, minerals, and antioxidants.

2. Sustain Physical Activity:
Engage in regular physical activities that bring joy. Strive for a blend of cardiovascular exercises, strength training, flexibility routines, and balance exercises. Consistent movement bolsters cardiovascular health, preserves muscle mass, and enhances mood.

**3. Prioritize Restful Sleep:

(3.)Sure, here are a couple of inspiring accounts of cancer survivors who reshaped their lives through changes in their eating habits:

1. Kris Carr: A Plant-Powered Transformation

Kris Carr, a renowned cancer survivor and author, faced a rare and incurable cancer diagnosis at 31. Instead of surrendering to despair, Kris seized control of her health journey. She embraced a plant-based diet abundant in fruits, vegetables, whole grains, and legumes. This dietary shift, combined with stress reduction, exercise, and mindfulness, played a pivotal role in Kris's transformation. Her story spurred her to pen "Crazy Sexy Cancer" and initiate a movement centered on wellness and empowerment. Kris's experience exemplifies how nutrition and lifestyle changes can facilitate healing and overall well-being.

2. Chris Wark: Drastic Diet Modifications for Healing

Chris Wark's journey offers another compelling illustration of the influence of nutrition on cancer survival. Diagnosed with stage III colon cancer at

26, Chris chose an unconventional path to recovery. He opted out of conventional treatments like chemotherapy and radiation, focusing instead on radical dietary alterations. Chris eliminated processed foods, refined sugars, and animal products from his diet, embracing organic fruits, vegetables, nuts, and seeds. He also incorporated holistic therapies and cultivated a positive mindset. Today, Chris is free from cancer and shares his story to encourage others to explore alternative approaches to healing.

3. Suzanne Somers: Integrative Path to Recovery

Actress and author Suzanne Somers encountered breast cancer and pursued an integrative approach to healing. Alongside conventional treatments, she integrated complementary therapies, including nutritional supplementation, detoxification, and stress management. Suzanne's dedication to nourishing her body with nutrient-rich foods, along with her commitment to holistic healing, contributed to her recovery. She documented her journey in "Knockout: Interviews with Doctors Who Are Curing Cancer," a book that delves into various treatment avenues, including nutrition.

These accounts underscore the transformative potential of nutrition and lifestyle changes for cancer survivors. Although each individual's journey is unique, these survivors' experiences demonstrate that taking an active role in one's health through diet and holistic practices can yield positive outcomes and inspire others to explore holistic approaches to healing. It's important to remember that these stories pertain to the individuals involved and that decisions about treatment and diet should be made in consultation with healthcare professionals.

Considering the interconnection of physical, mental, emotional, and spiritual well-being in achieving overall health.

These cancer-fighting foods are fortified with various nutrients, antioxidants, and compounds that have been the subject of research for their potential health benefits. Keep in mind that while these foods may have positive effects, maintaining a balanced diet, regular physical activity, and a healthy lifestyle overall contribute to well-being. Always consult with healthcare professionals before making significant changes to your diet, especially if you have underlying health conditions or are undergoing medical treatments..

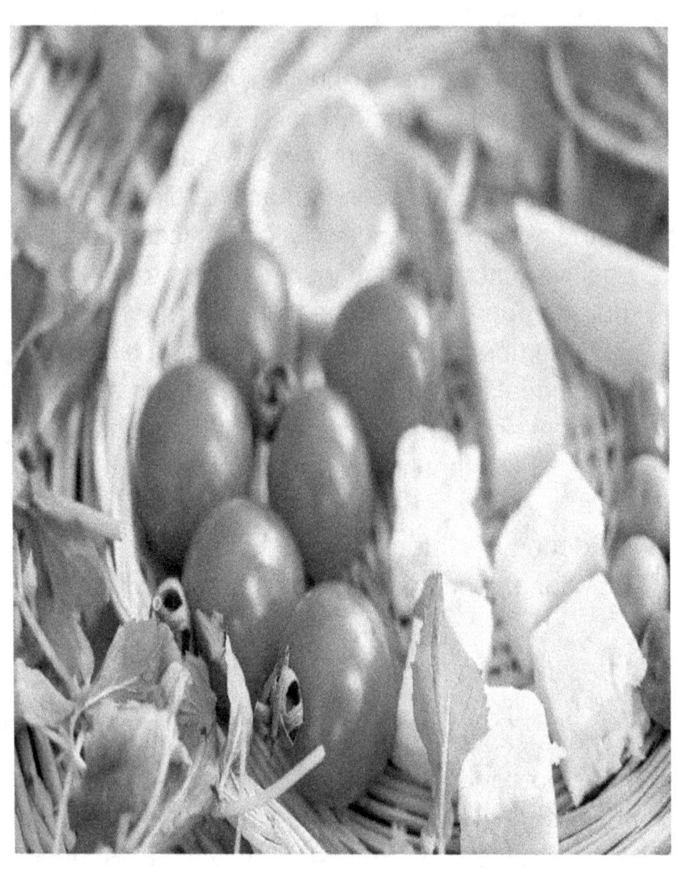

Conclusion

In conclusion, healthy food plays an important role in the battle to fight cancer. A well-rounded, nourishing diet has the potential to reduce cancer risk and help those in treatment. combining a mixture of fruits, vegetables, lean proteins, and whole grains into our meals daily,,it doesn't only boost our immune system it also build our bodies to fight cancer cells.it's necessary to remember that diet alone is not a miracle cure; it should be part of a large strategy for preventing and managing cancer, which includes regular screenings, physical activity, and adopting a healthy lifestyle. With the right nutriment and a total approach, we can make notable breakthrough toward a future with better protection against cancer.

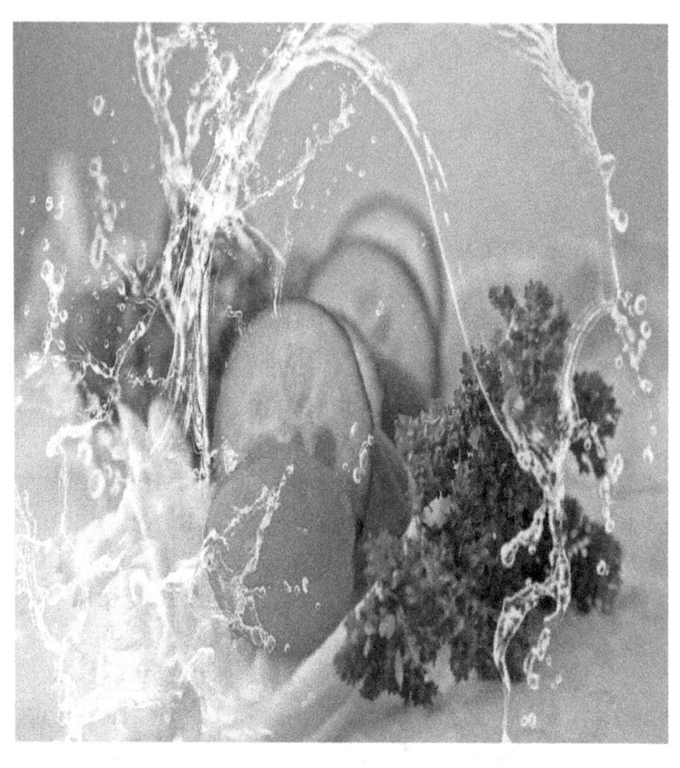

Daily Meal Remake

Day	recipes	Remake